The Body
of
Frankenstein's
Monster

The Body
of
Frankenstein's
Monster

Essays in Myth and Medicine

Cecil Helman

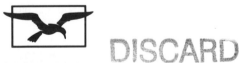

W · W · NORTON COMPANY
New York   London

ISBN 0-393-03104-7

W.W. Norton & Company, Inc.,
500 Fifth Avenue, New York, N.Y. 10110
W.W. Norton & Company Ltd.,
10 Coptic Street, London WC1A 1PU

1 2 3 4 5 6 7 8 9 0

To my daughter

CONTENTS

✧

Introduction   1

1 The Radiological Eye   13

2 The Body of Frankenstein's Monster   19

3 The Rise of Germism   29

4 Half-Green, Half-Black   48

5 The Premenstrual Werewolf   58

6 The Medusa Machine   81

7 A Bridge of Organs   94

8 The Dissecting Room   114

9 A Time of the Heart   124

Notes   140

INTRODUCTION

✧

This book is about Myth and Medicine, and about how, in a curious way, they both converge on the human body – or rather *bodies*, for there are many of them to be described here, all hidden within the same bulging bag of skin.

Among these many bodies is the magical body of myth and memory; the votive, sacrificial body; the body penetrated, but also impenetrable; the infected body; the invaded body; the bleeding body; the body damaged by devils and dybbuks; the body possessed by ancestral spirits; the archaic body of legend; the body in and out of harmonious balance; the body as disequilibrium and disease; the self-healing body of belief and trust; the body in time; the transparent radiological body, thin as celluloid; the modern, industrial machine-body; the hairy half-animal body, slave to the Full Moon; the sacred body of psyche and soul; the solitary, unknown, medical body; the shared body; the body crowded with autonomous organs; the dissected, dismantled body; and the fragmented, artificial body of Dr Frankenstein's monster – re-assembled by Science into an automaton of flesh.

All of these bodies are different, and yet somehow they are all the same, for they all revolve – like the spokes of a complex wheel – around the same familiar human form, staring back at us from the depths of the mirror.

One afternoon in late 1967, when I was still a medical student in the last year of my studies, some friends and I were sent to examine a middle-aged man, lying breathless and pale in a bed at the end of a hospital ward.

He was one of the dozens of patients that we examined over those few short weeks, frantically refining our clinical skills in the period before our final examinations. At first

1

glance there seemed to be nothing special about this man – but soon after, something very special *would* be happening to him, though at the time we knew nothing about it. A short time later his name would become famous, very famous, more celebrated than any of us would ever be. And his pale face too would be splashed across every newspaper and almost every television screen in every country of the world. For on that day, everyone knew him as the very first person to receive a human heart transplant, and as someone who – by living to tell the tale – personified one of the great triumphs of twentieth-century surgery.

And yet, to begin with, I was puzzled by the degree of media attention that the transplant attracted. For years, other organs such as kidneys or corneas had been successfully transplanted. Blood and plasma from one human body were daily being transfused into another, and artificial hips and heart valves had by then been implanted into tens of thousands of ageing bodies.

The answer lay not only in the technical brilliance or humane purpose of the operation, but also in the fact that the surgeon had somehow strayed into a mythic landscape, a land of signs and metaphors, where 'Heart' still stood as a universal symbol of emotion, courage, intimacy, and will.

Now for the first time one of the most important metaphors for personhood had been cut out, handled and cleaned, and then placed inside the body of another individual. In a few historic moments, the borders of one human body had been breached by the symbolic core of another.

For a while, after the operation, all those familiar idioms such as 'to take heart', 'with all my heart', 'from the bottom of my heart', 'a heart to heart talk' had a peculiar new salience, a double meaning both medical and metaphorical. During the operation itself the recipient was literally 'heartless' for that brief – and by now mythological – pause, as the surgeon lifted the old broken heart out of his body, and handed it to an assistant, before replacing it inside the empty chest with the healthier heart of another.

In this exchange, both donor and recipient had, quite literally, 'lost their hearts' to one another, via the matchmakers of medical science, so that afterwards, with his heart now 'in the right place', a man who had once been 'sick of heart' could resume his everyday life, as 'hearty' as before.

At the time, it had seemed to me that this heart transplant marked one of those great convergences (though by no means the first) between the world of medicine and that of myth and metaphor. For one dizzying, petrifying instant, the protective boundaries between Nature and Art, between physical reality and the language we use to signify it, were suddenly dissolved.

I had seen how fragile this boundary was, elsewhere in my medical studies, especially when dissecting human remains in the anatomy department. But a medical education made clearer in other ways the many links between language and flesh. Those famous lines in the poem by T. S. Eliot – 'We are the hollow men, we are the stuffed men' – had already had an uneasy resonance for me as I watched a man hollowed out during an autopsy, or when I peered through a body made empty and transparent by an X-Ray.

I was not surprised, some years later, to read in the press another example of how the metaphors of language could become, as it were, *embodied* in human flesh. It was when a totally artificial heart – a clever little device of pumps, tubes and valves – was implanted in the chest of an American patient, and his wife was reported as saying (apparently without irony) how relieved she was to find that he still loved her after the operation – and the kids as well.

In *The Cyclops* – a play from ancient Greece written by Euripides – Silenus, leader of the Satyrs, urges the Cyclops (he 'who eats his visitors and asks for more!') to consume

3

Odysseus, who has just landed near his cave on Mount Etna and has asked him for assistance. 'Swallow him whole! Eat every morsel up!' cries the Satyr to the one-eyed monster. 'And don't forget his tongue! That ought to be the medicine to promote loquacity!'

This enthusiastic suggestion, like the great excitement over the first heart transplant, makes sense against the background of the many metaphors with which we have invested the human body. Like the transplanted heart, the talkative tongue of Odysseus carries with it a heavy symbolic load, as one of the essential elements of 'humanness'.

Medical science, especially in its modern, high-tech form, often gives the impression that the human body has few secrets left to discover. Yet – though it has been penetrated by X-Rays, opened up by generations of surgeons, and had its cellular structure scrutinized daily by a multitude of microscopes – on some level the body still remains as opaque and mysterious to us as it always was. For, as Silenus pointed out to the Cyclops, the body has something more than a mere physical reality. It is more than just a collection of organs, cells and enzymes. For one thing, it has a unique relationship to language, existing as it does in the domains of narrative and myth – as well as being the repository of all sorts of metaphors for the human condition.

Modern language is as full of somatic metaphors as it was in Euripides' day. Some – like 'the Achilles' heel' – are taken from ancient mythology, while others are more recent in origin. To 'swallow one's pride', to 'get something off one's chest', to 'feel it in the bones', to be 'tongue in cheek', 'toothless' or 'spineless', or to have 'guts' or 'gall', are all bodily metaphors, which together constitute a special kind of 'body language'.

Late in the nineteenth century, in his studies of 'conversion hysteria', Freud pointed out other examples of the embodiment of metaphor. He described, for example, how hysterical patients, who were unwilling to 'swallow an insult' from another person, might develop constriction of the throat, and thus be 'unable' to swallow food or drink; or might get 'heart' pain if they had been 'heart-broken' in a failed relationship. According to Freud, their feelings had been converted into physical symptoms, subconsciously chosen for their symbolic significance to that individual.

I thought of this relationship between language and flesh – though in a very different context – when, as a medical student working in an urban slum, a man showed me a deep infected wound at the back of his calf. There was something unusual about that lesion, for I could see dozens of tiny black filaments protruding from it – almost like the spikes of a sea urchin – though the seas that surround the Cape were many miles distant.

No, the man assured me, the spikes were not those of a sea urchin; they were the hairs of his dog. He had taken that old adage – 'The hair of the dog that bit you' – literally, and acted accordingly. When his black-haired dog had bitten his leg, during a drunken mêlée two days before, he had chased and caught the offending animal, cut off some of its hair – and then rubbed it into the depths of his wound, as a hopeful form of cure.

Several years later, when I was studying social anthropology at London University, the story of the man with the hairy wound made more sense to me, as I came to appreciate the importance of myth, symbol and allegory in all human life, and to understand how they can influence both beliefs and behaviour.

In all societies, people live their lives in a sea of metaphor and myth, gathered together from many sources. Most of these arise from within their own 'culture', from the unique view of the world held by each group or tribe or society – a shared, inherited 'lens' of concepts through which the group's members learn to perceive, and react to, the world they live in. This culture is transmitted between generations largely by language, ritual and example. It provides people with ways of perceiving themselves, and their own bodies, and how they function in both health and disease. It offers a repertoire of concepts, words and images which helps each of them to organize, and to make sense of, the shapes of their body – as well as its symptoms and cyclical changes, the functions of its parts, and its relationship to other human bodies within the same society.

But it seemed to me that in the more complex, urban and secular parts of the industrial world – unlike more rural or religious communities – many of the allegories and assumptions that underpin our lives, and which we incorporate into our bodies and actions, could only be discovered in a more indirect way: perhaps by looking at the ways they are made manifest in the ideology and practices of our medical system, or in those oblique, but significant, corners of the modern imagination: advertisements, soap operas, children's books, and the cinema.

This new type of society – with its worship of machines, and clocks, and the products of industry – provides us now with a multitude of new images of the modern self – images as fragmented and kaleidoscopic as the milieu from which they arise. And it also provides us with new ways of talking about and understanding the body, new sets of models and metaphors for its moods and changes, which may be termed, collectively, our new 'body myths'.

Much of this imagery is borrowed from the artefacts of daily life. To 're-charge my batteries', 'to let off steam', 'to re-programme myself' or to have 'a nervous breakdown' are all metaphors gathered from the science and technology of the industrial age. But as I realized later, body myths are also drawn from a multitude of other sources, both old and new. And often they are a mishmash of contradictory elements, that echo the confusing mishmash that is life in the late twentieth century.

★

Because of my interest in the myths and metaphors of popular culture, one new source of body imagery caught my eye. It seemed to me that in this harsh, metallic era, the *cinema* – particularly its genres of 'fantasy' and 'horror' movies – offered us one of the last retreats for the mythic imagination of man.

Sitting in the velvety darkness, as our ancestors once clustered around their sacred shrines or campfires, our minds have gradually become populated by the characters and imagery of the silver screen. For several generations now, ever since the birth of the moving film, we have absorbed a new iconography – one filled with spirits and werewolves, vampires and monsters, with invisible invaders from Outer Space, artificial men and artificial women, and the destructive progeny of a hundred mad scientists.

But though the technology of cinema is relatively new, most of its images are somehow familiar. Often they take us back even beyond the fairy-tales of our childhoods – all the way back to the rites, myths and mysteries of our pre-industrial past. Slumped in the dark, and staring at that distant screen, they allow us to return along a celluloid road to a lost and legendary world, where ogres perish and witches flee, where Beauties and Beasts fall in love and marry, where everything ends happily in that final, satisfying moment when we rise to our feet as the lights come on.

Some of the *frisson* we feel, particularly in horror films – but also when watching a medical documentary – arises not only from the powerful feelings of *déjà vu* that they invoke, but also because there is something curiously 'contagious' about the images themselves.

Reflecting as they do some of the basic themes in modern culture, they tend to leak off the screen, and into our lives – and there is nothing we can do to stop them. Some people find they can use these images to conceptualize themselves and their own behaviour. Horror and fantasy films, for instance, offer us the idea of the human as half-animal (like the werewolf), as a collage of independent parts artificially joined together (like Frankenstein's monster), as a charming but fatally contagious lover (like Count Dracula), or as someone invaded by unearthly Aliens, or by Demons, or even – as in the movie *Fantastic Voyage* – by the microscopic technologies of medical science.

Behind its white-coated masks and scientific disguises, modern medicine is heir to many of the traditions and techniques of more archaic forms of healing.

Despite its emphasis on empiricism, its cult of numbers and objectivity, and the clarity of its experiments, much of its mythic and metaphorical content still remains – however impoverished. It is there if you look for it, hidden in the wide-eyed glances of its radiological eye; in its rites of diagnosis, dissection and treatment; in its worship of the diagnostic machine; and in its everyday use of the healing powers of belief, symbols, ritual and – above all – *narrative*.

Quite early on, I had realized that to be a doctor is to live one's life largely in a world of narratives, of tales and legends that are told and re-told many times over.

The folklore of medicine – its anecdotes and 'case histories', its ways of constructing and explaining the various types of ill-health – were already familiar to me, long before I entered medical school. Once, when I added all my relatives together, and then included myself, I realized there were no less than a dozen doctors in the family – as well as a few rural barber-surgeons scattered further back in the family tree. But it was only when I became a medical student, walking the long hospital wards, where each bed told its own story of suffering, that I fully appreciated the central role of stories and myths in medical care; and how, situated at the heart of every healing relationship, there could be found a series of narratives.

All illness and unhappiness generates its own, very special types of tale. This is because telling a story is one of the most basic human ways of organizing experience – and of shaping suffering into a form, in order to give it meaning. Over time each patient develops their own story, a personal creation added to and encouraged every day of their disease. Some grow into lengthy chronicles, or sagas, like those murmured on a couch by some thoughtful Scheherazade, as she tells her psychoanalyst – in One Thousand and One Nights or more – the sad story of her life.

In every culture, tales of misfortune form a unique genre, at once universal and yet personal and particular. These tales draw their imagery not only from individual experience, but also from the religion and culture in which they arise. Thus, in one place illness is couched in terms of 'possession' by spirits, in another in terms of divine punishment, or as invasion by invisible 'germs' or 'viruses' in a third.

Such stories have their own structure, and their own special sense of time and space. 'The pain began there on Tuesday,' someone may say, 'and then it moved to here on Wednesday; now at the end of the week, it's all over my body.' Seated on the distant side of the doctor's desk, the patient gestures here and there, outlining in the air the map of a mythic country, populated by suffering and pain.

As he listens carefully to the patient's tale (which medicine calls 'the History') and then moves forward to examine him, the doctor finds himself lost at first in this unfamiliar landscape of symptoms and signs.

But as he travels further, gradually probing the surface of the riddle and its hidden interior, he begins to recognize along the way certain place-names and direction signs, certain one-way streets and cul-de-sacs. Slowly he begins to understand the internal syntax, the underlying pattern of all those many symptoms and signs – here the cadence of a voice, or the hue of a skin, there the texture of a tongue, the droop of an eyelid – until finally he is ready to decode the true message, the one that lies deep within the patient's discourse, hidden in the labyrinths between its words.

★

Now at last it is time for the second narrative – the turn of the doctor to tell his own earnest tale, to recount a story of exploration, discovery and future plans. Scribbling on the pad before him, he describes to the patient his own complex journey of diagnosis, and what he has discovered along the way. He tells him what has happened, and how, and why, and what should be done to make it all better again. And as he talks, he begins to describe – and prescribe – a future in which his needles, drugs or scalpels will enter the very organs and cells of the patient's body, introducing into its biography a new story with many possible endings, some of them happy, others not.

Just as medical diagnosis involves the constant process of turning the body from flesh into metaphor, so medical treatment seems to consist partly of turning metaphor back into flesh.

All of this is occurring daily – in hospitals, clinics and doctors' offices, as well as on radio, television, and everywhere else that people gather new sets of narratives to mingle with their own.

In the process, something subtle and unusual is happening to our bodies, something invisible, and yet affecting us all. Slowly and surely, under the influences of science and the cinema, of modern medicine and advertising and technology, people are acquiring a new set of conceptual bodies, a different way of describing their physical and emotional experiences. Gradually they are turning into anthropomorphic machines, into the oracles and idols of medical science, into assemblages of independent organs and the borrowed parts of other bodies. They have become porous to invisible invasion by germs and viruses – just as they were once vulnerable to possession by the spirits, devils and *dybbuks* of a distant past. In the centre of their newly transparent chests, the hearts of these industrial bodies now beat to the cadences of the industrial clock, and the metronomic rhythms of urban life.

But although many of these changes are happening all around us, as well as within us, they cannot be fully described either in the dialects of medicine, or in those of the social sciences. It seems to me that they can only be adequately portrayed in the realms of metaphor, in a new language and in a new type of narrative – as fragmented and mythic as the new body itself.

CHAPTER 1

✧

The Radiological Eye

There are four luminescent panels in the room, in a silver frame on the table, and rows of black books on a shelf, and journals, and crushed styrofoam cups with the barnacles of yesterday's coffee. Rectangles of X-Ray film are pinned to the panels, a dark parade of skulls and skeletons in the underwater light of the little room, in the white-tiled building with many corridors. This is the radiology room, the room of white bones and empty flesh.

It is almost a century now since Wilhelm Conrad Röntgen discovered the invisible X-Ray, and at the end of 1895 published his monograph – *Eine neue Art von Strahlen* ('On a New kind of Rays') – in the German city of Würzburg. A few days earlier, on the 22nd December, in a moment of medical history, he had passed these new kind of rays right through his wife's opened hand, and then onto a photographic plate.

We can still see the ghostly outlines of Frau Röntgen's hand, with the dark finger bones and the large oval ring, and still they throw their long shadows over our perceptions of the human body. For the first time the eye travels to within the living body, and peers around inside, without ever tearing open its envelope of skin. The body is transparent now, and because of that some part of the mind, too, loses its solidity and becomes more permeable to the outside eye.

★

The aim of radiology is still the uncovering of secrets, the revelation of mysteries that are masked by flesh. With the aid of radiology you can 'see through' or into someone, but their selfhood is dissolved by your gaze. Look at the screen now, and there is no one there. All that remains of the individual are the imperfections of form: a broken bone, a swollen heart, a twisted womb, a back hunched over like a question mark. The human beings have all disappeared, shrunk to the banal cartoons of Hallowe'en. Stare at these too long and even they will vanish, as the bones weaken, and the cells of the marrow become malevolent and multiply.

But now look a little closer at the screen, for seen through the radiological eye your body can encode all the cycles and seasons of the year. Within the human frame the rays reveal a natural landscape of light and shadow, a chiaroscuro of suffering or health. It is a paradoxical world, a world turned inside-out and upside-down. The topographies of skin and expression have gone, so have all the solidities of organs, and muscles and tendons. Only their spectral, translucent shadows remain on the screen, still outlined in skin.

In these shadows we can recognize the echoes of midnight or noon, autumn or spring. There is the clear summer light of a healthy limb or lung, or the little white flakes of infection scattered over a dark chest, like a snowfall at the beginning of a winter's night.

There is the 'rib cage', as it is called, with its most famous inmates: the pulsing boot-shaped heart, the long conduit of the oesophagus, the spongy irregular lungs, and the large blood vessels arching backwards to behind the heart. In radiology, as in language, here in the cage is the heart of the matter, the seat of metaphor. Here is the universal flesh-box of the emotions, and within it – whether hard, soft, warm or cold, broken or black – vibrates that little personality, hidden within the Self.

In this *mundus inversus* of hidden forms, the hollows of the body tell their own story. It is a text of spaces and absences, of empty shapes that are filled with meaning, like the plaster casts of vanished corpses in the hard larva of Pompeii, or the shadows left on the rocks of Hiroshima. Together, the dark body and its empty crevices form a fragile unity, a Jungian fusion, whose only imbalance can be sickness or death.

In the iconography of a life, X-Ray plates are unwelcome guests in any photo-album, or box of portraits or holiday snaps. But the X-Ray is also a photograph, though of a poignant and particular kind. Like other photos it is only a fragment of a bigger story, only a rectangular slice of time, a split second in the trajectory of a life.

The writer Susan Sontag has noted the native surrealism of the photographic art, and how it relies on 'the very creation of a duplicate world, of a reality in the second degree, narrower but more dramatic than the one perceived by natural vision'. But in this novel reality, context is everything, and much of the meaning lies in the narrative. The tale told about the holiday snap surrounds it like a frame, and gives it a meaning. There in the telling is the feel of sunburnt skin, the full stomach, the mosquito bite, the sound of cicadas from behind the castle, the smells of the ocean or the scent of bougainvillaeas. But the story told of a radiograph, in square white hospital rooms, is sparse, and therefore mysterious: only a name, a date, a number, a diagnostic phrase, and always hovering somewhere in that room, an invisible human being.

But in other ways, X-Ray plates are a truer chronicle of the human moment. The random snap encapsulates the photographic past as well as the spectator's present, but the radiograph reveals more than just the biography of a body, and the labels given by the medical gaze. It is also a true photograph of the future, a snapshot of the skeleton inside waiting to be born, the one still hidden in its womb of flesh.

This parade of photographic skeletons and skulls, glowing on the screens of the radiology room, reminds me always of

El Día de los Muertos, the Mexican fête of the dead. This is their All Souls' Day, an heir to the ancestor worship of the Aztecs, which takes place every autumn throughout Mexico. It is like a festival of the radiological eye. On this day skeletons of wood, plaster or papier-mâché are displayed, wearing bright everyday cloaks and sombreros, some carrying flowers, or wine, or musical instruments. Each is a *memento mori*, a grinning messenger to the plump and the unconcerned. In the early dawn light, families trek to the cemeteries, taking with them candles, tiny sweet skulls and skeleton candies, and ample offerings of flowers or food. They hold picnics near the graves of their relatives and, sitting on the ground, as one traveller has written, 'they tell and re-tell stories of the dear departed whose death they have come to mourn, and whose virtues they wish to perpetuate.' After the picnic the uneaten food is left at the gravesite, as a posthumous feast for the dead. For this one magical day, a singular hole in time, there is a communion between the worlds of the living, and the worlds of the dead. The masks of life are stripped away, and the family members of both worlds share a meal across that transparent wall – thin as an X-Ray plate – that still divides them.

If you inject opaque dyes into the hollows and channels of your body, or drink them down deep into your crevices, then the white shapes on the X-Ray screen will paint a ghostly Rorschach inside your body.

For radiology reminds you that man is hollow. He is merely a doughnut, a bagel of flesh. You can outline the tortuous tunnel passing through this Hollow Man from his mouth down to his anus, with the creamy white liquid called Barium. Swallow a cupful, and as it waterfalls down the long tube of the oesophagus, you can see on the X-Ray screen some of the mythological possibilities of the human body.

There in the chest is the spinal column, with its twelve branching ribs, like a white Tree of Life in the centre of a

16

Garden of Eden. In the lower part of the Garden, below the Tree, rest the two serpents of the bodily myth. The fat white worm of the Colon, its outline sketched in Barium, belches and stretches under the low hills of the diaphragm as small shudderings of peristalsis move the pellets of food along its length. And beneath it is the other serpent, the convoluted one, the Small Intestine, with its sluggish curves and crenellated back.

Elsewhere in the body, dye coursing through arteries and arterioles shows, as if from an aerial view, all the branching streams and tributaries of great, broad rivers flowing throughout the body. All the four rivers of Eden are there, Pison, Gihon, Hiddekel and Euphrates, with their forks and tributaries, their wandering brooks and tiny rivulets.

Now pour dye into the thick tubes that carry the vital air into the lungs, as they branch out from the windpipe into the 'bronchial tree'. See the ever-narrowing branches of this Tree of the Knowledge of Life fill with dye, and form a white and delicate bonsai, its feathery web of twigs and boughs bare for the winter. Notice how sometimes this tree carries on it a deadly fruit. The dye avoids an irregular area in the bonsai: instead of whiteness, there is a small black hole, a 'filling defect' on the film. A tumour has been found. Now a fatal Apple hangs from the branch, ready to poison the peace of the Garden.

To the West and to the East, multifaceted stones lie scattered in the kidney and its drainage tubes. They are curiously shaped and sculpted, as if fashioned into the hard idols and obelisks of an obscure, microscopic culture. North-West of them lie clusters of tiny stones in the globular gall-bladder, like piles of pebbles forgotten on a beach.

Inject a dye into a vein in the arm, and the kidney excretes it into the urine. It flows through the two thin ureteric streams, from their stunted baobab openings in the kidney, down South to the pale oval lake of the bladder. In either direction, in the flanks of the Garden, a renal arteriogram

17

reveals how in each kidney the blood vessels divide into an intricate tracery of tributaries – a Nile delta of tiny streams and rivers on either side of the body.

Here, in the newly transparent human form, an enigma repeats itself. Radiology has assembled the pieces of an ancient puzzle. The elements of the jigsaw, some old, some new, are all there on the screen: a shadowy Garden of rivers and hills, two Serpents, a white branching Tree of Life and one of Knowledge, a Cage, a line of Idols, and there – glowing in the very centre of the Garden – a lone pulsating Heart.

CHAPTER 2

✧

The Body of Frankenstein's Monster

The big figure in a darkish suit moves slowly and clumsily across the shadowy screen.

We stare at him as, like some huge and hydrocephalic child, he lumbers through the cardboard streets of the little village of Golstadt, under the clouds of a celluloid sky. We see in close-up that he has indeed the face of a brutish child, but with something also of the physiognomy of the intellectual about him – the tall bulging skull of the 'egg head', or the 'high brow'.

This is the figure whose allegorical footprints are imprinted deep in the clay of our modern mind, in the visual folklore of the age.

We recognize its face, its irregular walk, those mournful and cavernous eyes, the terror that stomps with heavy shoes among the cinema crowd.

It is that familiar monster of Dr Frankenstein.

The story takes place somewhere in a Germanic Central Europe, in a landscape of feudalism and fear, a land of small stone villages and the lonely castles of remote aristocrats. Superstitious peasants shamble about their business, and through the camera's eye we peer down at the wary squint of their locked faces, under the shadows of narrowing streets and alpine hats.

19

In this film, the writers of Hollywood have re-created in fantasy the peasant past of their ancestors. It is a Europe of the mind, a mythic blend of longing and amnesia. An image blurred at the edges, like a fading daguerreotype, or the memory of something lost in childhood.

Vaguely the spectator is reminded of those other map references in our modern collective unconscious – the Carpathian Mountains, the roads of Transylvania, the wily peasants, the frightened Burgomaster, the man in the cloak, the old castle crumbling like a broken tooth at the top of the hill, the screams that echo through the fog.

We learn soon of the diabolical hubris of/Dr Frankenstein, of his plan to create a new life out of the fragments of death. With his quick gestures and efficient features, he is the epitome of the gentleman scientist, the educated amateur, a sort of early industrialist, his laboratory a factory for the production of a New Man/

Born in this womb of metal and glass, his monster is a collage of pieces of the dead, fragments of a dead past sutured together with twine, and animated by the powers of science and electricity. 'That body is not dead; it has never lived,' says the doctor. '*I* created it. I made it with my own hands, from the bodies I took from graves, from the gallows, any-where.'

Like Voltaire's *ingénu* or poor Kasper Hauser, the monster is an adult child, a violent, bewildered toddler born suddenly into a hostile and incomprehensible world. Even the actor Boris Karloff saw the monster he portrayed as essentially innocent, 'a pathetic creature who, like all of us, had neither wish nor say in his creation'.

But there is an error in its design. By mistake, a criminal's brain has been transplanted into its skull. Like all those other offspring of male procreation, the monster is a clumsy, violent and inarticulate being – just like those armies, states, bureaucracies, computers and cars, given birth to by man, just like that bomb named 'Little Boy', the one whose howls of hunger obliterated in moments the entire city of Hiroshima.

Together, Frankenstein and his monster form a total Gestalt, a unity of selves. Creator and creation are two halves of the same being, cold intellect twinned with brutal force. The scientist has given life to his offspring, and even his name, but for all its violence it is the monster and its tragic fate that earn our attention, not its maker/ Born at the beginning of the film in sparks of electricity, we know that it must also die in fire, destroyed by an enraged peasantry in a singular *auto-da-fé*.

But the monster's demise is only temporary. It awaits rebirth in the next film, and in each of the seven sequels made by Universal Studios. In the thirty-two Frankenstein films, made between 1910 and 1976, the monster dies again and again, and yet each time is reborn in a celluloid reincarnation. But even as each new generation of monsters appears, the grand icon of the genre still remains the version of 1931, with its melancholy chiaroscuro, and Boris Karloff as the doomed monster.

The films are based loosely on *Frankenstein*, Mary Shelley's epic novel published in 1818, and subtitled *The Modern Prometheus*. Far beyond the imaginings of its author, her book has laid seeds that were to germinate in another time, in other continents, and which flower in our consciousness even to this day. The book narrates how the Swiss, Victor Frankenstein, creates an artificial man, assembled from human fragments gathered from charnel houses and the 'unhallowed damps of the grave'. By the use of an arcane science, he is able to 'infuse a spark of being' into the lifeless thing. As it grows into self-awareness, its cry: 'Who was I? What was I? Whence did I come? What was my destination?' forms the poignant core of the novel. But the experiment is doomed to a tragic dénouement. The monster, driven to a

21

despairing rage by the rejection of mankind, destroys all who are close to its creator. Let Man 'live with me in an interchange of kindness', it pleads in vain, 'and instead of injury I would bestow every benefit upon him with tears of gratitude at his acceptance'.

The story ends in gothic style, with Frankenstein dead, punished like Prometheus for his perverse provocation of the gods, while his creation floats remorsefully away on an ice floe, exulting in the freezing death to come.

Like all those other horror films – of Dracula, the Werewolf, the Aliens from Outer Space – the Frankenstein films recapitulate, in cinematic form, ancient mythological themes from our European past. The Scientist, the Assistant, the Laboratory, and the Monstrous Creation, have all become the ciphers of a modern myth, which itself is a palimpsest of more archaic themes. Here we can recognize echoes of an earlier mythology: of Prometheus' challenge to the gods; of the Creation of Man; of the myths of birth, death and rebirth; of the destructive tension between parent and child, creator and creation; of the perpetual ambiguity of innocence; up to the modern 'mad scientist', and his cold indifference to human values.

Furthermore, the monster is truly the son of man, the product of male procreation alone. Its creation by Baron (or rather 'Barren') Frankenstein is a pitiful imitation of woman's fertility. 'If Dr Frankenstein was, in a sense, the father of his creation,' wrote one critic, 'then lightning was its mother.'

This myth of a purely male procreation, often from natural materials, has an ancient provenance. In Genesis, God created Adam from earth, but then Adam's flesh gave birth to Eve. In Greek mythology, Hephaestus created the giant Talus from bronze, on the island of Crete, and Pandora from water and clay. The sculptor Pygmalion made a woman from ivory, and then fell hopelessly in love with her pale nakedness. In the thirteenth century, the Necromancer

Albertus Magnus, known as Doctor Universalis, is said to have made a living man of brass, though some still say it was made of bones and of flesh. In the sixteenth century, the physician and alchemist Paracelsus, in a perverse parody of female fertility, created a little homunculus by incubating his own sperm for forty weeks in a pile of horse manure. And about that time too, Jewish legends tell of the Golem, a man made of clay – just like Adam – who was created in the ghetto of Prague, and then animated by the power of holy words, until one day it ran amok.

And there is another archetype that takes root here: the myth of the modern 'mad scientist', with his wild white hair and bulging, unfocused eyes. For Dr Frankenstein has a long literary and cinematic genealogy, numbering among his fictional ancestors and recent kin the notorious Dr Jekyll and his shadow self, Mr Hyde; Dr Moreau, the creation of H. G. Wells, alone on his island of man-made animal-men; Dr Xavier, creator of the terrible Moon Monster; Dr Cameron, maker of werewolves; Dr Strangelove, crippled lover of the atom bomb; and old Dr Caligari himself, with his big locked cabinet of terrible secrets.

Anthropologists and historians have noted the curious reciprocity between our images of the personal body, and those of the body politic. We see society as if it were an organic body, and the body as a sort of society of organs and parts. Each may come to symbolize the other. We use the imagery of one to explain the workings of the other. And this is true, too, of fictional bodies, like that famous body of Dr Frankenstein's monster.

For this grotesque body, part now of the iconography of our time, symbolizes also a new type of society, and its novel powers of destruction.

It is a purely male society, violent and inarticulate, that emerges against a background of feudalism and peasant life. It is a collage of ancient elements, gathered from different

23

pasts, and sutured together within the same body politic. It is animated by science, and by electricity, but it has the brain of a criminal. It meets rejection and hostility from the people around it as it stomps among them, and tries to destroy them in turn. But at the end it dies in a chorus of angry screams, at bay among its enemies, in the roar of firestorms and of buildings crashing down in an iridescent shower of sparks.

In the 1930s and in the decades after, there is a clear resonance between the world inside the dark cinema and the darkening world outside: between the images on the screen and the rise of dictators, the world at war, the explosions, the burning buildings and the chaos, the industrialization of genocide, the atomic bomb, and the lumbering 'arms race' between competing 'war machines'. On the screen walk the huge metal monsters of war, crushing village after village under their enormous feet. And there are the familiar faces of the mob, the flaming torches, the loud cacophony of screams, the peasants in their *lederhosen* gathered around the piles of burning books or people. The monster and its destructiveness are the only possible progeny now, of the mind of a criminal mated with the cold rules of logic.

Frankenstein's dream of an artificial man is also dead, but the dreams of *partially* artificial men have now been reborn in the 'spare part' surgery of modern medicine, in the widening use of *transplants* and of *implants*. In the late twentieth century, new bodies, a new society and a new sense of self have been created by the new generations of Dr Frankensteins.

Transplant surgery creates bodies which carry within them the organs or tissues of *other* bodies. 'Man falls apart, piece by piece,' writes a surgical textbook, and 'transplantation is designed to replace exhausted parts as they fall.' The recipient is now a walking collage of the living and the dead. Within him there are kidneys from close kin, and heart and corneas, liver and lungs, cartilage, skin, hair, bone, nerves, lymph nodes, pancreas and parathyroid – all from the bodies of dead strangers. Bottles of blood, plasma and bone marrow donated by other strangers, drip–drip into his veins, and into the veins of the aged and the ill.

Transplants create an original kind of kinship between recipient and donor, both living and dead. In a secular world, this produces a type of partial immortality. For when a man dies, his kidney can live on. Heart, liver, cornea and blood become the names of his descendants. Billions of his cells will continue to live, planted like seeds in another man's body.

In the age of transplants, what was non-self is now self. The boundaries of human skin have finally been breached, as the bodies of the aged and the ill dissolve piecemeal into one another.

There is now another new body. Like the new society in which we live, it is a temporary assemblage of industrial parts, a soft and moving machine clothed in skin. This is the other half of 'spare part' surgery, the world of implants.

Now there are prosthetic organs of plastic, metal, nylon and rubber. There are artificial heart valves and bones, synthetic arteries, corneas and joints, larynx and limbs, teeth and oesophagus. There are machines implanted inside the body, and outside on its surface. The heart beats now to the electrical rhythms of a tiny pacemaker. There are hearing aids and iron lungs, dialysis machines and incubators. In this century, a new body has been born, an ancestor of the *cyborgs*, those advanced fusions of man and machine that Alvin Toffler predicted would one day occur.

The body and its implants create a new way of organizing society, new networks of need between the self and others. Somewhere out there are the shadowy thousands who make, market, repair and maintain these artefacts, or who shape and package them, as well as all the many surgeons, technicians and nurses who implant them.

In our brave new productive world the body, like society,

is seen as an organized machine, and the machine itself just as a hard-edged human. We can all become a temporary assemblage of parts, our boundaries pierced by sculpted implants, and the tissues and organs of other people.

The parts that wear out can now be replaced, for capitalism demands the notion of replaceable parts, as well as replaceable people. The ageing body, once part of industry, is now part-industrial. The worker retires, old and tired after years working in a factory, but the factory reclaims him. He becomes a novel type of consumer, displaying the products of medical industry on the shelves and sideboards of his very own body, and a living advertisement for their efficiency.

In this world of urban fragmentation and anomie, there is a sense of a shrunken self, of a tiny homunculus crouching deep inside us, surrounded by borrowed organs or plastic parts.

These brand-new parts of people are impersonal, mass-produced, and stronger than the rest of the body. Many of them will outlive the flesh in which they are implanted, for, like transplants, they promise a temporary piece of eternal life, a partial life beyond the grave.

One day puzzled archaeologists will sift, frowning, through the dusty gravesites of our culture. On the glass shelves of their great museums there will be no arrow heads or pottery or jade jewellery, but rather steel hip joints, plastic arteries, ceramic teeth, a metal heart, and a row of hearing aids.

Both new body and society are constructed from different elements from the present and the past: some living and contemporary, some industrial and mass-produced, others ancient and traditional. The society is created not by one Dr Frankenstein, but by many, and with the aid of nuclear as well as electrical energy. Its language of xenophobia, and its discourse on immigration, mimic many of the physiological processes of 'spare part' surgery. For in medical theory, the body's 'defence system' deals ruthlessly with any 'invasion' by 'foreign bodies', such as grafts or microbes, and these invaders may be 'rejected' by the 'host', and attacked by its 'antibodies' or 'natural killer cells'. Only those grafts most similar to the body – the organs of very close kin – are easily 'accepted' by the body, without such a violent 'hypersensitivity' reaction.

Thus in a similar way, immigrants and refugees, those quintessential 'foreign bodies' transplanted uneasily from country to country, may also encounter a range of receptions from their 'host' communities – rejection, hypersensitivity, or even sometimes a reluctant 'acquired tolerance'.

Implants, transplants, cyborgs and neomorts have all been predicted in popular myth and culture, in science fiction and the horror film. From *The Golem* films of 1914 and 1920, and the famous *Frankenstein* of 1931, up till *Coma*, *The Hands of Orlac*, *The Bionic Man* and *RoboCop*, they carry many decades of warning about the dangers of artificial men, of mechanical societies, and the rise of anthropomorphic machines.

Karel Čapek's play *R.U.R.*, of 1923, where the world is taken over by sinister robots created by men, is a pioneer of this genre, and so is Fritz Lang's film *Metropolis*, made in 1926, with its harsh images of industry, its allegory of robot bosses and their robotized proletariat. Among the more recent descendants of these early robots are HAL, the ruthless, flat-voiced computer of Kubrick's *2001*, and the more whimsical robots whirring along the deserts of *Star Wars*.

These films blend images of a new type of society with those of the new types of bodies, manufactured of metal or flesh, that now live within them. But the celluloid creation of artificial man is no longer the preserve of fiction or fantasy. For twenty years or more, in the medical documentary film, art, nature and surgery have all blurred and dissolved into one another. Organ transplants and organ implants are news now, and their operations high drama. The *cinéma vérité* of medicine, with all its blood and silver scalpels, flickers often over the living-room walls. Famous transplant surgeons flit across the television screen, their Colgate teeth glittering on talk shows, their eyes aglow in the quiet light of the operating theatres.

And lying there silently on the bed, we see the covered form of a 'neomort', brain-dead and comatose, as he waits for his organs to be harvested, and floats like a balloon between the two great Worlds, still tethered to us by the tubes of a life-support system.

Regularly we greet on the television the recipients of these transplants or implants. Dozens of them smile and wave at us from the screen, their grateful, chubby faces bloated with cortisone.

The medical documentary is the new genre of social realism, but one which is curiously familiar to us. We pass through the rectangular doorway of the television screen, into the world of the super-hero scientist, in the midst of his eternal battle with the shadowy forces of Time, Age and Disease. The cone of our attention converges on the knife, the suturing hand, the moist transplanted heart, the electrical defibrillator held just above it. There is something familiar, a Technicolor feeling of *déjà vu*, about the swathed figure on the table, the shining glass and metal, the crimson blood, the tall scientist and his humble assistants.

The viewer watches as this drama unfolds, and waits. Somewhere, as the heart leaps suddenly into life, he listens for that triumphant cry of Dr Frankenstein, the proud yell of the new parent, that has echoed from the screen into the foyers of our minds, ever since 1931 – 'It's alive!' cries the mad Doctor. 'It's alive!'

CHAPTER 3

✧

The Rise of Germism

It is only a little pamphlet, called *The Common Cold: Relief But No Cure*, published in 1976 by the United States Department of Health and Human Services, but there on the cover is this panoramic view of a frantic 'cold war', of a violent battle between tiny homunculi and their mortal enemy, the Germ. These germs or viruses are portrayed as tiny devils with forked tails, their little faces twisted into a hairy snarl. As we watch them they are flying around the page and swooping up and down through the embattled air, flinging their pointed lances, and stabbing here or parrying there. The troops of Health are fighting back. They use tanks, planes, artillery and bottles of cough mixture. They shoot pills, capsules, bullets and missiles at their enemy. Soon some of the little germs are shot, while others disintegrate. The smells of cordite drift through the air. The battle spills over onto pages 2, 4 and 6 of the pamphlet, but the devilcules are everywhere – tiny, hairy, invisible things, waiting in ambush. For the moment their tide has been halted, but the War goes on, as it will always go on, for ever and ever.

Meanwhile, on the other side of the Atlantic in Britain, the official Health Education Council issues a pamphlet – *Germs are a Dirty Business* – for those handling food. 'Just a moment's forgetfulness', it sternly warns, 'can be a germ's opportunity' . . . 'there's not a part of your body in which germs won't congregate and breed' . . . 'Germs hate heat,

29

but love the warmth' . . . 'heat and humidity create the very conditions in which germs flourish' . . . 'a sick person is a natural carrier of germs'.

These two images – tiny devil, and invisible but ubiquitous peril – have ancient roots in Western culture, as they have elsewhere. Today we call their descendants 'Germs', but in the modern world these entities have become metaphors, as well as microbes. For germ infection is among the dominant images of the twentieth century, and it incorporates many of the moral mnemonics of our time.

In the everyday use of the term, 'germs' have become a potent symbol, embodying within them a whole cluster of meanings and memories, of ways of being and ways of interpreting many of the phenomena of everyday life. This lay, metaphorical use of Germ Theory, taken out of its original medical context, is what I would term *Germism*. Its origin lies in a collage of folk traditions and diluted science, in bits of bacteriology blended with magical thinking. It is a way of talking, but also a way of thinking – a set of beliefs, perhaps even a sort of folk religion, whose images are drawn from the discoveries of Pasteur, Koch and Lister, but with only a slight understanding of scientific cause and cure.

Germ imagery is subtly woven into modern language, and into the fabric of colloquial speech. It is common nowadays to speak of 'an infectious laugh', of 'contagious joy', or 'a catchy tune'. The headlines of the popular press warn daily of the 'virus of soccer hooliganism', the 'epidemic of muggings', or the 'rash of bankruptcies' that seem to afflict us. And daily they urge action against the 'plague of terrorism', and all the other crimes and violence 'endemic in our society'.

This imagery of contagion – unseen, and yet disruptive – has spread to include the material objects around us. Even that metaphor for the modern mind and the reliable brain – the computer – has now fallen victim to its own, metaphorical infections, and to unseen invasions by 'software bugs' or 'computer viruses'.

The writer Susan Sontag has described how in the past diseases of uncertain origin could sometimes become metaphors, crucial carriers of social and moral meaning. In the nineteenth century, grave diseases such as cancer, cholera, syphilis and tuberculosis became such metaphors, and to an extent they are still today. They were images 'awash with significance' of the moral wrongs and postures of human society. For many in the nineteenth century, tuberculosis – with its pale and delicate victims – was at the core of a romantic world-view. It was believed to result from a heightened sensibility, coupled with a lowered vitality, and became a fashionable disease among the poets and literati of the day. Cancer, by contrast, was believed mainly to afflict bitter, isolated people, full of repressed emotion that made them vulnerable to a sort of 'demonic possession' by cancer's 'malignant' or 'primitive' cells.

But the germ infections of today are very different from nineteenth-century tuberculosis and cancer. For one thing, they are no longer of such uncertain origin. With the aid of science we can see, measure and even count the germs as they strut across the circular stage of the microscope slide. For that is where they were first spotted, as far back as 1683, when the Dutch scientist Antoni van Leeuwenhoek saw them through the crude microscope that he had invented. But it was only in 1859 that Louis Pasteur in Paris showed the world that these unseen beings actually lived in the air, and were all around us. Then in 1882 Koch tracked down the infamous Tubercle bacillus, and Klebs showed us the Diphtheria bacillus the following year.

Since then we have learnt much more about these tiny organisms. In the modern world, a vague knowledge of 'germs', their habits and their hobbies, is part of our popular culture. Despite this, for most people the idea of 'germs' still remains a hypothesis, a theory of causality, a way of explaining the inexplicable. For how many of us have actually ever *seen* 'a germ' under the microscope? And besides, even if you do peer down its long metal tube, the enigma of the germ remains. There are no little devils there on the slide. Only tiny spheres stained pink, purple or a darkish blue – some of them bunched together like grapes, others laid out in long serpentine chains, or scattered over the slide like a child's marbles across the living-room floor. Or you can see clusters and fans of rods or spirals, or little swimming things with fast undulating tails and slim flagellae.

Magnified many thousands of times, their power is still mysterious to the modern eye. How can such tiny toys, such little crayons or balls or sticks, cause fever or pain? How can this pink sphere, or that innocent red spiral, fester a mind, or slaughter a body?

Yet somehow these puzzling and invisible agents do enter unseen. They seem to possess the body like an evil spirit or a *dybbuk*, and cause misfortune or death. Like a sperm or a seed, they are implanted inside you, to 'germinate' over time into a symptom or a disease.

It is curious how people speak of germs as if they were singular, as a solitary 'my Germ', 'your Germ', or 'his tummy Bug'. 'I've picked up your Germ,' someone says, 'I should have been more careful.' For in this age of individualism, even germs have a right to their own name and personality. In the modern metaphors of Germism, these personalities are woven into the passage of time, into the slow revelation of a specific cluster of symptoms. Like possession by devils or spirits in other cultures, you recognize them, not by what you can actually see – in the air, or under the microscope – but by the revealed symptoms and stigmata of their presence within the human body.

'I've got the one that gives you the dry cough and the watery eyes,' they say in the suburbs, or 'the one that gives you the rash and the runny nose', or the measles, or the mumps, or the one that devours your nerves, your brain, or your liver. Silently the germ seems to enter your orifices, silently it swims along the bloodstream, spreading to your organs. And then suddenly when it is ready, it declares its presence by a fever, a pain, by phlegm or catarrh. Now to fight against it you must 'feed a cold, starve a fever'. In the folklore of 'flu, if you rob the hungry germ of its food it will surely starve, or fly away.

In the imagery of Germism, most infections are seen as social events, for they always imply another person. They seem to occur at the points where people's lives intersect with one another. At these crossroads of human behaviour, if one person is the victim of an infection, then another must be its 'carrier'. The germs are believed to pass invisibly between them, sometimes jumping from skin to skin, sometimes flying through the air, or carried along on their breath, or even leaping out of a smile. Different types of encounter seem to contain within them different types of germs, from the quick, moist infection of a lover's kiss, to the slow ripening of a venereal glance.

Thus, woven into Germism, there is the idea of the porous self – of a self open to penetration by an invisible 'something' that originates in other people. Over many years, this image of contagion has subtly shaped how we understand the mind and its emotions. It has given us models, borrowed from bacteriology, of how the emotions of one person can influence – one could even say 'infect' – those of another. For just as you can 'catch' or 'pick up' the virus of another person, so can you also 'catch' their 'contagious joy', or their 'infectious laugh'. The negative emotions in particular – such as anger, envy or fear – are often spoken of as if they were microbes – immaterial pathogens that somehow fly through the air between people (especially between parent and child), striking one of them down with hurt, guilt or even illness.

Some of these ideas, influenced by Germ Theory, about

the effect of people on one another, also echo those of advertising, education and propaganda. In each of these perspectives, invisible influences – both ideas and emotions – are also believed somehow to 'enter' the mind, through the open doors of its perceptions, and to plant their permanent seeds in its fertile, subconscious soil. A conscience, a memory of trauma, a prejudice, a collection of historical facts, the loyalty to a group, a product or a leader – all of these obey the idiom of an unseen entry into the mind and body, and their final germination over many years into the varieties of social behaviour.

On a more solitary level, some choose to explain the flux of their own emotional life in a bacterial idiom, but in the language of infection from elsewhere. In this particular view, the borders of the mind are described as permeable to outside penetration – by moods, ideas, thoughts or reflections – originating not within other people, but from somewhere 'out there'. Unpleasant emotions or moods seem to enter the self at will, and then set up their residence within it. 'Six months ago, following a bereavement,' writes a correspondent in the London newspaper *The Independent*, 'I stumbled out of a long, dark winter infected with depression. It had invaded my body like a creature from outer space, making me a zombie among the living.'

In everyday talk, the words 'germs', 'viruses', 'bugs' and 'bacilli' are often used interchangeably – lumped together as if they were all the same thing. In this pervasive metaphor there is no place for 'good germs'. For since last century germs have been seen as always evil, though science knows of millions of so-called 'normal flora' – the tiny bacilli who live in peaceful coexistence with the skin and membranes of every human body.

Despite this, the Germ Theory of modern medicine – and its noisy step-child named Germism – have always carried with them the imagery of war, of attack and counter-attack against an unseen enemy. In 1906, in a celebrated speech, the scientist Paul Ehrlich had described how medicines 'able to exert their final action exclusively on the parasite harbored within the organism would represent, so to speak, magic bullets which seek their target of their own accord'. Since their discovery during World War Two, it is the antibiotic drugs that have become these magic bullets, the germ-seeking missiles of medicine. Every day they are deployed on that mobile field of battle, the human body. On all sides (and not only on the covers of government pamphlets), a 'germ-warfare' is being waged by the doctors, and a war against those who harbour these germs, especially those foci of 'low resistance' – the poor, the weak, and the morally inept.

The Age of Germism dates from about the days of Pasteur, in the middle of the last century. In Europe and in North America this has been a time of hot wars, and cold wars, and of massive social changes. The world of the nineteenth century seems to have turned itself upside-down, and around, and never returned to order again. Even in the past half-century, men have flown to the moon and back, others have swapped their hearts for new hearts, nuclear bombs have exploded, millions have fled into the huge electrical cities, and the great empires of the world have crumbled away. For many now living, the Age of Germism has seen the decline of religion, and of much of its explanatory power, while in its place have flourished the cults of Science and of Medicine. Now as they diffuse into the population, the models of medical science offer us – in a distorted, diluted form – a set of secular metaphors, a collection of symbolic tools for making sense of this complex and unpredictable world.

This Germistic way of thinking places the blame for our misfortunes on powerful, capricious 'forces' that are said to rule over our lives – just as they were once ruled by devils, or by Divine grace or punishment. Nowadays we call these shadowy entities by different names. They are known to us as 'market forces', or 'inflation', or 'high interest rates', or 'nationalism', or 'the people's will'. As forces of change they are often just as malign and invisible, but much less personalized than their tiny, contemporary cousins, the 'viruses' and the 'germs'. Over many years, these two images – malign 'forces' and malign 'germs' – have gradually become blended together, creating a blurred picture at the periphery of our modern consciousness. It is a collage of old ideas and new images, of shadowy, disruptive pathogens lurking in the corners of our everyday lives, and waiting there to destroy us.

Because of this, the Germistic way of thinking always implies a sense of passivity, and of helplessness. For who can control which 'germs' will choose to enter our bodies, and fly in through our orifices, or when this will happen, or why? And who can really control which 'forces' will wreck or enhance their lives, and who can do much about pollution, radiation and unemployment, or the 'ailing economy', the 'sick pound', or the fearful 'epidemics' of crime they say are spreading throughout society? As with the microbes of 'flu and tuberculosis, we seem to be the innocent victims of obscure forces, of events that lie far outside our own control.

The idea of germ invasion, and the spread of infection, is above all a metaphor for *sudden* social change, a signal of acute moral uncertainty, sometimes of chaos. The anthropologist Mary Douglas has appropriately called dirt, 'matter out of place'. In the Germ Theory of modern medicine, the clear relation of dirt to infection is symbolic, as well as actual. For in our infected and changeable world, the 'dirt' of disorder seems to be everywhere. Much of the sense of order and continuity has now become the 'matter out of place' of the contemporary world. Year by year, the certainties of thought and behaviour are seen to be breaking down. In this transient and entropic world of civil unrest, and the shifting fads of the consumer society, Germism provides us with a way of describing these changes – talking about them in a language of serious, unexpected infection. For like a revolution, a riot, or an economic crisis, a powerful bacillus can quickly undo the structures of a human life, undermining its postures of rank and of power. In their infirmity, the adults can become child-like, the powerful are debilitated, the prince and the pauper cough up the same khaki phlegm, the rich vomit like the poor. In the sickroom that is modern society there is fever, phlegm, vomitus and pus. For germs are a dirty business, and their liquid dirt and stigmata of disorder are all about us, leaving a dark stain on the ordered cosmos of bourgeois life.

Like our ancestors before us, we try to preserve the fragile order of our lives against these invisible threats by using spells and talismans to repel them. We wear lucky charms, fine-smelling herbs, crucifixes, Saint Christophers, Stars of David, packets of garlic, and pieces of bright-coloured cloth pinned to our clothing. Some of us – the devotees of science and of medicine – use pills and vaccines and antibiotics and all the other inner talismans of medical science. In our homes there are shrines, ikons and protective mottoes, and finally – but only when all else fails – there are slim insurance policies, hidden in the cupboard.

In political discourse, 'germs' have become the symbols of other, uncontrollable influences – of invisible forces that invade the borders of the state, rather than those of the self. For the Germistic world-view is essentially xenophobic. It is a world of boundaries, and also of the fear of those boundaries, and their inherent fragility. Hidden in the metaphors of germ infection there is a fear of the penetration of that conceptual skin between self and non-self, between them and us, that brings with it the dread of chaos and moral contamination. In the popular press, immigrants and

37

foreigners are often blamed for importing these moral infections, and are themselves seen as metaphorical germs, infecting and invading the body politic.

The xenophobic eye sees waves of such infection immigrating in from beyond the known and ordered world: from Africa, the Caribbean, the indecipherable East. It watches as Eastern influenza viruses launch their annual mass attacks on the bodily and ideological citadels of the West. Wave after wave of 'Asiatic 'Flu,' 'Red 'Flu', 'Hong Kong 'Flu', 'Taiwan 'Flu', come and go. Each year there is a wait for these ruthless, alien germs, their tiny faces twisted into that familiar snarl as they throw their lances and swamp the 'defence systems' of body and state.

In the late Roman period, at the birth of Christianity, almost all misfortune was ascribed to invisible, suprahuman agents called the *daemones*. The air of Byzantium was dense with these ubiquitous, malevolent forces. Even sorcerers could only cause harm by manipulating them.

Two scholars have written of the world-view of those times. 'If we believed that the myriad bacilli about us were each and all inspired by a conscious will to injure man,' they wrote, 'we might then gain a realization of the constant menace that broods over human life in the biographies of the Byzantine saints.' It is odd how, since the days of those early saints, so little has changed in our perception of invisible dangers; Antoni van Leeuwenhoek and his discoveries seem to have passed without trace. Most of the world has hardly peered into his long brass microscope, and it remains puzzled even when it does so. On some level we still prefer our invisible devils and their personal malevolence. Under the masks of science, many of us still live in Byzantium.

Every day this seems to become more true – right here in the world of modernity, among the flickering of computer screens and all the high-tech horrors of industry and war. On all sides – warn the media pundits of newspaper, radio and television – there are pervasive perils and invisible dangers.

The air in the Greenhouse in which we live, they say, is stuffy and thick, filled with radiation and ultra-violet light, with pollution and lead. There can be no relief for us from the cool radioactive rain, or the acidic dew, or the wind that carries the factory fumes from over the hill. The clear spring water you drink may well be impure, your food is probably a fatal collage of chemicals and colours. There is penicillin in the meat, mercury in the fish, and an allergy floats in the bottle of milk. Invisible rays seep out of the walls of houses, and into your body; they creep out of watch dials or radios, out of microwave ovens and television sets, to soften your bones and rot your skin. Everywhere in the air float unseen gangs of malevolent germs, sauntering through the streets on the breath of innocents, turning to attack us at random. Who can save us now from these invisible perils? The priests are confused, the doctors evasive. Night after night the myopic scientists look even more pensive on the television screens. Who can trust them any longer, or believe in that wry smile of modern medicine, with its knives and nostrums, its piercing rays and thalidomides?

In this modern motif of a poisoned and phobic planet, the germ – like the *daemon* before it – has come for some to symbolize unpredictability, 'bad luck' or 'fate', and all the chaos at the margins of the conceptual world. In this modern version of an ancient myth, the modern *daemones* seem no less capricious than their ideological ancestors. Why do they strike here, and not there? we ask. Why does this person get infected, and not that one? Why does one person rot from radiation, and not another? 'Why me? Why now?' cries the victim. 'What have I done to deserve all of this?' He feels innocent, but also vaguely uneasy. There is something ambiguous about his position. Perhaps, after all, he did transgress. Perhaps he remembers that infamous decree of the judges in the witch-trials in Salem, Massachusetts in 1692, declaring that 'the devil could not assume the shape of an innocent person in doing mischief to mankind,' and that those possessed by Satan were always guilty. Perhaps there is something careless or immoral about him too, to make him vulnerable to those dark forces at the periphery of the ordered mind.

The sick man wonders whether somehow he has broken the laws of self-care, and been possessed by the secular *succubi* and *incubi* of the germ world. Perhaps he is now contagious, and a threat to the innocents around him. Who knows whether – like those whose necks carry on them the rabid lovebites of Count Dracula – he might yet carry the contagion of evil with him in his every act, in every whim or gesture.

Writing of that long-ago devilry in New England, Marion Starkey notes how irrelevant it was that none but a few young girls could actually 'see' the devil himself, and so point the finger at his accomplices. After all, bacilli today are just as invisible to the naked eye, and for the worried burgers of Salem 'the girls were the microscopes which God Himself had provided for the laboratory work of detecting witches.' It was all a fearful experiment, carried out *in vivo* in the New World, and as the busy witch-finders searched for the answer, the innocents swung in the gallows' breeze.

In Salem, as in the mass European witch-hunts of the sixteenth and seventeenth centuries, they stigmatized the old women and the marginal men, the crippled and the ugly. These were the suspected carriers of moral contagion. They 'diagnosed' them by signs, by their curious sighs, by arcane portents on their skin or limbs. They knew them by their blemishes, by the matter out of place on their bodies, by the 'Devil's mark' hidden under their skin. Or sometimes, during the trials and torture, they saw it by the message written into their bodies, in the unfolding of their satanic symptoms

— in the sudden emergence of gruff cries, or mad writhings, or twisted spasms of terror.

In many cultures outside Europe, *spirits* are believed to cause disease, but there is compassion for the victim, and not a sentence of death. The anthropologist I. M. Lewis has described several African societies where illness is blamed on possession by 'disease-bearing spirits'. Among the Luo people of Kenya, for example, disease and other misfortunes, whether trivial or severe, are blamed on amoral, malevolent spirits of external origin that possess their victims in a capricious, unpredictable way. Among followers of the *bori* cult of the Hausa people of Nigeria, each spirit – like its Western equivalent, the germ – is associated with a particular cluster of symptoms, such as fever, pain, cough or bleeding. And like germs, these living, invisible spirits seem especially to attack the weak and the poor, though members of the cult believe that their cure is by exorcism, and not by antibiotics.

Unlike many of the devils of Europe, these African disease-spirits are amoral and largely disinterested. They strike without rhyme or reason, arbitrarily infecting either the innocent or the guilty. Misfortune is so random that the victim is considered blameless, and can easily gather a caring community around him.

Elsewhere in the world, the individual is not seen as a victim, but rather as a willing host of these spirit invaders. The *shaman* – that charismatic folk healer of many traditional cultures – allows the gods or spirits to enter and possess him, to fill his soul with their power, and during a trance to talk to the community with his voice. So do mediums, diviners, healers, channellers, and the practitioners of glossolalia, those speakers of unknown tongues. Somewhere deep inside themselves, they believe, a living and sentient force is allowed in as a temporary guest, until after the seance, or the ritual of healing.

★

In totalitarian or closed societies, the repertoire of social action has often been drawn from medicine and its Germ Theory, and the rhetoric of politics from the language of bacteriology. Built on harsh hierarchies of fear and repression, the exercise of power in these societies often takes the form of a 'treatment' of the 'sick' body politic. To the presidents-for-life, dictators and caudillos, dissent and free thought are often seen as dangerous bacilli of the mind. For they conceptualize ideas as 'germs', as invisible and contagious influences that pass from person to person, flying through the airwaves, or diffusing from the pages of books, or wandering through the ether from ear to ear.

In this variation of the Germistic world-view, some people are themselves seen as 'germs', or at least as the contagious carriers of such germs. Dissidents, rebels and artists are treated as if they were the vectors of such infection, implanting their intellectual microbes – perhaps even the 'germ of an idea', the idea of freedom – as they move secretly among the people.

In 1865, the surgeon Joseph Lister realized, from the writings of Pasteur, that wound infections were not caused by 'dirty' air as many had thought, but by the tiny organisms carried within it – and that the air around the patient could be 'cleaned' of these organisms with a special carbolic spray. In the totalitarian societies of today, Lister – like Pasteur before him, and the more recent discoverers of antibiotics – has become the unwitting author of social laws, of modalities of social 'treatment' by the political versions of antisepsis, hygiene or quarantine. For such models of medicine fit easily into the schemes of modern dictators, dedicated these days to the more 'scientific' control of their captive populations.

To those regimes who use the metaphor of the 'sick society', infected by enemies from without or within, the air in the political sickroom will always be polluted. It can only be cleaned of the invisible germs of dissent and agitation by a vigorous spray of political carbolic. Or by applying the rules of antisepsis, by washing out the brains of their victims, or killing their carriers by genocide, deportation, or by 'starving a fever'. Or by quarantining those carriers – by the use of house arrest, or imprisonment, or banishment to some distant and septic Siberia. Or by controlling the spread of their idea-germs by censorship, or blank newspaper pages, by the burning of books, or the jamming of broadcasts. Or by applying the aseptic, hygienic techniques developed in the 1870s, to prevent germ infection in the first place: by the practice of *apartheid*, by erecting Berlin Walls of the mind, *cordon sanitaires* between pure and impure thought, and by guarding the orifices of the nation with watch-towers and dogs, with barbed wire and machine-guns. Or even – most drastic treatment of all – by killing all those infected by the germ, one by one, in a deserted courtyard one evening, with a magic bullet through the back of the neck.

The history of human conquest is often also the hidden history of a particular microbe, and from this they still draw much of their symbolic power.

Microbes were unwitting weapons in the Spanish conquest of the South American Indians, from the sixteenth century onwards. First there was smallpox, and then measles, and then typhus and influenza all brought in by the conquerors, and again in the seventeenth century, malaria and yellow fever imported with the slaves from Africa. A hundred and twenty years after the conquests of Cortez and Pizzaro, the Indian population was down by over ninety per cent. The great empires of the Aztecs and the Incas had fallen, not to the swords and musket balls of the conquistadors, but to invisible, genocidal germs carried within their bodies.

In Europe too, the invisible scythes of bacteria have swept across the continent's history, and their half-healed wounds can still be seen in its collective memory. Most terrible of all those bacteria was the one called *Yersinia pestis*, carried by rats, squirrels or mice, and also by tiny fleas nestling among their short spiky hairs. This was the bacillus of the Black Death, the terrible plague of the fourteenth century. It began in October 1347 in the harbour of Messina in Sicily, when a fleet of Genoese galleys docked, carrying with them plague victims from the shores of the Black Sea. Landing in port after port along the Mediterranean coast, from Italy up to France, the galleys spread the infection even further, till the plague covered the entire continent, killing millions as it swept from country to country. 'It was so contagious,' wrote Guy de Chauliac, an eye-witness of the plague in Avignon in 1348, that people caught it 'not only by staying together, but even by looking at one another.' As they fell seriously ill, some spitting blood, others with high fevers and swollen bubonic glands, 'men died without attendants, and were buried without priests. The father did not visit his son, nor the son his father. Charity was dead, and hope was crushed.'

Again and again over the next three centuries, the plague returned to Europe, though each time in a weaker form. Tens of thousands died during the Great Plague of London in 1665, but by the next century the epidemics had almost disappeared. Only in 1918, during the great 'flu epidemic, did a gruesome echo of the Black Death reappear, when over 20 million died in a world already debilitated by war.

Susan Sontag has noted now epidemic diseases, such as the plague (or 'pestilence' as it was once called) are usually conceived of as a disorder in the social fabric. 'Pestilential' in the Middle Ages meant 'morally baleful or pernicious', while 'pestilent' meant 'injurious to religion, morals, or public peace'. Such epidemics were seen by the people as signs of inner disorder, cruel symptoms of a deep moral pollution. The community was seen as being under mass attack by unseen powers, and scapegoats had to be found. In the fifteenth century some flagellated themselves for their unwitting crimes, others blamed the Jews as carriers of these evil spirits, and massacred them in 1348–9, just as Hitler did centuries later, after blaming them for 'spreading a moral tuberculosis among the nations'. Almost five hundred years were to pass after the human and bacterial massacres of the Black Death, before the *Yersinia* bacillus was found, and identified on a microscope slide, and then the culprit flea four years later.

Even today, the word 'plague' remains with us as a metaphor for chaos, social disorder, the terrors of uncertainty, and the sweeping punishments of a community's crimes. Media pundits and politicians still describe civil unrest, economic crises, crime and divorce, as if they were waves of infection, now reaching 'epidemic proportions'.

This way of thinking lies at the very core of Germism. For it places the origin of all social evil in *contagion* – as if it somehow arises outside the behaviour of 'normal' people, or of their leaders. But seen through the narrow lenses of Germism, the 'germs' said to cause these epidemics can never be identified. Nor can the problems they cause ever be solved. For as a moral model of the universe, Germism is a limited perspective on the complexity of life. Using the impoverished models it has borrowed from bacteriology, its insights are limited by its constant imagery of war and attack, by its relentless search for invisible enemies and scapegoats, by its ignorance of economics and the structure of society, and by the meagre slices of life visible to it on the microscope slide. Most dangerous of all, it can only explain the flux and complexities of social life by inserting tiny, conceptual devils into its hypotheses – and then by blaming them and their 'carriers' for all our social ills.

The solutions that Germism offers are just as limited: merely more and expensive magic bullets, aimed at all those inexplicable modern influences which – like the *daemones* of the past, and the hidden devils of *Yersinia pestis* – have caused terror by overturning the certainties, piercing the boundaries,

45

and bursting through the walls of both mind and state.

In the last quarter of the twentieth century, the modern equivalent of the Black Death is AIDS, the Acquired Immune Deficiency Syndrome, the 'gay plague' of the screaming headlines. In a way, it is the apotheosis of Germism, a symbolic fusion of the human body and the body politic. Like cancer or tuberculosis, it has become one of the most powerful metaphors of the age. In the discourse of the popular press and television, the AIDS virus is described as if it were an invisible and alien invader, crossing the borders, infiltrating the cells, and weakening the 'defence systems' of body and society. It is seen as a hidden force, one that undermines society's 'resistance' to social disorder and to invasions by other germs, spirits, or malevolent devils.

The medical response to this 'invasion' by AIDS, like its response to other 'germs', is couched in the imagery of war. It is a World War, waged against a cunning, invisible, ubiquitous enemy. But this battle with the new Germ-man is not only against a deadly virus, but also against its bearer, the homosexual, and other carriers of subversive sexuality. Homosexuality itself is now conceived of as if it were a virus, a contagion to which the innocent and the young have little resistance.

But the metaphors of AIDS are as unique as the century in which they appear. With the decline of the Cold War, they are gradually evolving into something new – into the imagery of a global guerrilla warfare, or a low-level counterinsurgency, a viral Vietnam rather than the mass battle imagery of the Wars on Crime, Cancer or Drugs. Increasingly, the AIDS virus is described in terrorist terms, as if it were a hidden enemy attacking the weak and the unwary, slipping unseen with its bombs and grenades through the flabby moral defences of Western civilization, then into its organs and bloodstream.

So the AIDS epidemic of today and the ancient fear of unseen influences that it invokes, brings us back, right through the full circle of Germism, to the tiny flying devils and their lances, to the world of dirt and malign *daemones*, through the Black Death to the witch-trials of Salem, Massachusetts, and returns us finally to the new 'Devil's marks' of our time – an HIV antibody in the blood, or a Kaposi's Sarcoma hidden in the skin.

CHAPTER 4

✧

Half-Green, Half-Black

The story is apocryphal, but somehow true.

It goes like this: an anxious woman patient is given regular prescriptions by her doctor for a certain well-known tranquillizer – a little capsule which is half-black and half-green in colour. One day she tells the doctor (in some versions it is a relative or friend): 'Usually I take my capsule at bedtime with the green end first, and it works just fine. I have a long deep sleep, and I wake up rested and relaxed the next morning. But last night, for some odd reason, I swallowed it down with the *black* end first. And then it didn't work at all, and I had awful insomnia. I was up half the night tossing about, with nerves and panic, and palpitations too.'

A certain enigmatic power seems to be condensed into the green end of that little gelatin capsule – an invisible power that originates not in the medication, but in the woman herself. It consists, above all, of the healing, soothing strengths of her own mind, and of her belief in herself and in others – a belief so powerful that it can cure the body, and calm the mind. Projected onto one half of the tranquillizer capsule, it is the phenomenon that modern medicine now calls the *placebo effect*.

Whether it is a pill or a potion, almost anything you believe in can become a placebo. In medical practice, placebos are usually pills made entirely of sugar, or capsules that are empty inside. Although they look authentic, and have a convincing taste, they are really counterfeit drugs, cunning and plausible copies of the real thing. It is solely the patient's belief in their power and function that turns these inactive substances into a powerful medicine. But the placebo effect can also be found elsewhere – hidden, for example, in the healing powers of a smile, or a touch, in a gesture or a word, or even in the intricate rituals of a diagnostic test.

Research has shown how all manner of ailments have been helped by a belief in placebos. They are reported to have relieved angina pectoris and pain, helped hay fever and headaches, suppressed several types of coughs, lowered high blood pressures, healed ulcers in the stomach and the duodenum, and soothed the aching throb of rheumatoid arthritis. Many depressed, nervous and insomniac people – and even some schizophrenics – have been helped by the placebo effect.

Sometimes its unusual power can lie hidden in the actual shape, colour or name of a remedy or medication. Studies have shown how some tranquillizer tablets coloured green have calmed the nerves of anxious patients, but not when those same tablets were coloured yellow; while other scientists have shown how some depressed patients felt happier after swallowing down a yellow tablet, but not when that tablet was crimson or green. And certain headaches, too, have only been helped by pain-killing tablets when a famous brand-name was printed on their packet, but not when that packet was unlabelled and plain.

But these many types of placebo are not only healing in their effects – for they can cause discomfort, and even dependency upon them. Tell some suggestible people that they will feel weak or dizzy, impotent or ill, from a little pill made entirely of sugar, and some of them surely will.

Thus the placebo effect, with its many names and actions, and the many masks on its hundred faces, is part of a very powerful magic – the universal magic of belief. Its mechanism is mysterious, and its origins obscure, but in the long historical drama of human healing, it has always been the leading actor.

Friedrich Anton Mesmer, born in 1734 near Lake Konstanz, was the son of a gamekeeper, and a student in Vienna of the uncomfortably named Fr Maximilian Hell. He was a qualified physician, and the holder of no less than four doctorates, one of them in astrology. In later years he moved on to Paris where, under the patronage of Marie-Antoinette, he wrote his long and rambling *Dissertation on Animal Magnetism*. As a fashionable faith healer in pre-Revolutionary France, he became one of the most famous practitioners in history of the art of the placebo effect.

All of the universe, believed Dr Mesmer, was composed of a unitary and ubiquitous gas, which he termed the 'aestheric continuum', and which he claimed was dominated by the forces of magnetism. Any disturbance in the delicate balance of these magnetic forces of the universe, often under the influence of a disordered mind, could cause human suffering, disease and even death.

His famous trances of healing took place in a large room lined with stained glass and mirrors, overflowing with flowers and incense, and filled with the sounds of soft music. In its centre stood a large tub full of iron filings, with iron bars protruding from its side. Rows of wealthy patients sat in silent expectation around the tub, clasping each other's hands, or gripping onto the ends of the iron rods. Suddenly a slight *frisson* would ripple around the room as the great 'magnetist' himself entered, dressed in a lilac silk robe, and carrying in his hand a special iron rod, held aloft like a wand. Slowly he would pass around the circle, staring fixedly into each of their faces, while making arcane, mathematical movements with both of his hands – until at last, in a rustle of silk, a circle of swooning ladies would sink slowly to the floor.

In this way, many of his patients' ailments were healed by his invisible 'mesmerism', including the several forms of hysteria, as well as various pains and paralyses, convulsions, blindness, and even 'congestion' of the liver and the spleen.

It was an age in France when the tinderboxes of revolution were already beginning to spark. In this incendiary atmosphere, a puzzled Louis XVI convened a panel of experts – not to study the social unrest gathering around him, but rather to examine the curious cures of Dr Mesmer. Among the members of this panel were Benjamin Franklin, Lavoisier and the soon-to-be-infamous Dr Guillotin. By 1784 they had sceptically concluded that most of the cures were not caused by Mesmer's 'animal magnetism' as he had claimed, but solely by the suggestibility of his patients. That was the end of the matter, but there was a curious addendum to their report: 'It is impossible not to admit', they said, 'that some great force acts upon and masters the patients,' and that this invisible force 'appears to reside in the magnetiser.'

What was this mysterious 'great force' that resided in Dr Mesmer, and what is it now – two hundred years later? Above all, it is the magnetic charisma of the healer's personality, which in every generation needs for its power a potent placebo-blend of mesmerism and faith, as well as a ritual milieu of healing and care. It arises always from the centre of an ancient matrix of human beliefs – beliefs in the workers of wonders and miracles, in faith healers and holy waters, in magic cures and in magic curses, and in the healing touch of the Seventh Son of a Seventh Son.

Phineas Parkhurst Quimby, a famous and flamboyant faith healer born in 1802 in New England, and – like Mesmer – bearer of another 'great force', once put it thus: 'I tell the patient his troubles, and what he thinks is his disease, and my explanation is the cure. If I succeed in correcting his errors I change the fluids in the system, and establish the patient in health. The truth is the cure.'

Quimby's 'truth' is thus the universal self-assurance of all healers, from psychoanalysts to shamans: their belief in their own explanations, and in their metamorphic power over matter and mind. Everywhere, in their clinics or temples of healing, the main task of their many techniques is to shape, mould and give *meaning* to the raw clay of human suffering – to somehow order the turmoil of their patients' perceptions, the terror of disorder, and the chaos of fear. Around all of this they erect a scaffolding of reassurance, an intricate cage of concepts to which only they have the key.

Over the centuries, wise doctors and traditional healers have always seen themselves as the allies, and not the enemies, of the healing powers of the self. They have seen their task as cooperating with all those remedies concealed in the brain and the blood, as working with the shamans of the white blood cells, and the logical gurus of the immunological system.

Yet though many healers have shown how belief can heal ulcers, soothe pain, lower the blood pressure, and calm a frightened brain, the placebo effect still remains as the uninvited and invisible guest at the celebratory banquets of modern medical science. In textbooks and in journals, its curious power encounters only the collective sneer of the medical profession. There it is described as '*only* the placebo effect' – not as a 'real' drug or effect, but '*just* a placebo'. It is still spoken of by most of the medical world as if it were only a bogus and confusing element, merely a false phenomenon in the smooth machinery of high-technology healing.

Yet somehow, despite all of this, it still remains as an enigmatic gap at the centre of the rational paradigm of modern medicine. Right there, in the very heart of medical theory, there is a numberless, unpredictable and uncontrollable void. But look more closely at the shape of that void, for over the years the sneers of science have seeped right into it, and filled it up like plaster in a mould. Slowly as it sets we recognize its familiar shape, the curious symmetry of its bumps and projections, the emerging limbs, heart, nose, eyes, ears, ideas and memory, and hear – from somewhere within it – the faint sounds of a human voice.

It is Act One, Scene One. A doctor's office, somewhere in the Western world, sometime this century. It is a clean, hygienic room, with a faint bouquet of expensive disinfectant. There are bright fluorescent lights on the ceiling, and a framed diploma hangs on the wall. Shining instruments lie scattered on the shelves of a glass cabinet, like the iron rods of Anton Mesmer. On another shelf stands a double row of plump textbooks, their Latin names lettered in gold.

Gathered behind the doctor's desk are the ancestral portraits of legendary doctors, a gilt-framed genealogy that stretches all the way from Hippocrates, Galen and Maimonides up to Pasteur, Harvey and Sir William Osler.

In the corner of the office there is a wash-basin, a square of shining tiles, and a pair of clean white towels hanging from a rail.

Now there is a tentative knock on the door. Slowly it opens, and an anxious patient enters the room, and glances around him. A man, or a woman, rises smiling from behind the large cluttered desk with a hand outstretched. The doctor wears a white coat, or a smart grey suit, and his silver spectacles are worn over a mask of detached benevolence. Around his neck hangs the two-headed serpent of Aesculapius, each of its plastic mouths waiting to whisper its message into his attentive ear. A beeper and a golden row of pens stand stiffly to attention in his pocket. On the desk lie a silver ophthalmoscope in its box, and three cardboard obelisks of medical files.

As he takes his seat at the centre of this theatre of medical magic, the patient inhales deeply of the heady, disinfected air. Somewhere deep inside himself, a frightened child creeps into the early morning warmth of its parents' bed.

He looks around the room, and as he does so his eye

gathers together the mystical ciphers of the power of Science, forming them slowly and calmly into a grammar of belief. Now he takes another, and deeper breath, and then, with a sigh, begins to speak . . .

The doctor's office, like Mesmer's great room of flowers and incense, or the crowded halls of Phineas Quimby, is a sort of secular Lourdes, a shrine to the faith of the cities and suburbs. Here, like the guru in his long limousine, or the shaman in his fur and paint, he supplies the pieces missing from our personal jig-saw, and ritually re-assembles the broken fragments of our humpty-dumpty world. In this familiar ambience of healing and trust, the charisma of his power surrounds all of the drugs, both real and placebo, prescribed for his patients, and coats them thinly with an invisible layer of belief.

Wrapped in this ritual envelope, the tranquillizers or sleeping tablets that his patients carry away with them become a symbolic tonic, fuel, food or friend, at the very centre of their impoverished lives. The bottles of bright-coloured antibiotics that he dispenses become the medical 'magic bullets' fired at their enemies, those tiny Germs or Viruses hidden somewhere within themselves. While all those hundreds of heart drugs, pain-killers and blood-pressure tablets so regularly prescribed, weave themselves slowly, day by day, into the ordered fabric of patients' lives – and there become the emblems of their disability, their magnets for empathy, and the circular metaphors for their doctor's love.

Like the black end of the tranquillizer capsule, there is a dark side to the placebo effect. It is the harmful, pathogenic effect of both belief and trust, and is called the *nocebo* effect – from the Latin *noceo*, I hurt.

The most awesome example of this effect – the killing power of a public curse – is the phenomenon anthropologists call 'voodoo death', 'hex death', or even 'magical death'.

They tell how it has happened in Africa, Australia, the Caribbean, and elsewhere. There is something of the stuff of horror films about their tales – the sort that flicker on the television screen on a wet winter's night – or of the wild recollections of elderly travellers.

On the cinema screen, its usual image is that of the voodoo priest, a dark man squatting near the flames of a midnight fire, as he rummages among the entrails of a decapitated rooster. Beside him on the hot Caribbean earth lie the little manikins of wood or of wax, pierced all over with pins. Several scenes later (and here the hairs begin to rise at the back of our necks), we hear those familiar, irregular screams as they echo among the rows of little wooden shacks, and watch as the camera pans past the faces of the terrified crowd, and then sinks down slowly towards the victim – the man found dead and goggle-eyed in his bed, with not a mark on his petrified body.

This is the familiar nocebo of Hollywood, the fatal power of a celluloid curse – but in the canons of true anthropology, although the dénouement is often the same, the picture is much less dramatic. In that same heat of the tropical air, a certain man realizes that he is doomed, cursed publicly for a particular crime or moral transgression by the words of a powerful priest, witch, shaman or sorcerer, acting on behalf of the tribe. Slowly over the next few days, his clansmen and kin withdraw from him, shaking their heads, and avoiding his eyes. 'Shortly thereafter,' writes the French anthropologist Claude Lévi-Strauss, 'sacred rites are held to dispatch him to the realm of shadows. First brutally torn from all of his family and social ties and excluded from all functions and activities through which he experienced self-awareness, then banished by the same forces from the world of the living, the victim yields to the combined terror, the sudden total withdrawal of the multiple reference systems provided by the support of the group.' The man is now socially dead, an object of fear and taboo, his corporeal self merely a shadowy hallucination in the eyes of the tribe. Shortly thereafter, his

55

body too will die, in an expected and yet mysterious way.

Some years later, though many thousands of miles away, and far from the tropics, an old woman is torn away suddenly by her children from her tiny room, her little shrine of memories. Against her wishes they place her in an Old Aged 'Home' in another city, in a huge and anonymous building that can never be her home. And very soon afterwards she too dies, suddenly and mysteriously, and is found cold and staring in a little room bare except for a bible, a torn nightdress, and a brace of family photographs that stare silently through her from the bedside table.

And meanwhile, elsewhere in that same distant city, a white-coated high priest or sorcerer enters a hospital room, and with the needle of a sterilized syringe pierces a certain patient's body here and there, peers through it with a special machine, and then rummages for an answer among those medical entrails of paper and celluloid – the patient's blood test results and his X-Ray plates. The doctor in the white coat looks down at the sick man and then, slowly and gravely, he shakes his head. With a swallowed sigh, the patient's friends and kin gathered around the bed mumble their excuses and then leave the room, one by one. Something invisible happens to the patient then, when he is alone again – something final, cellular and microscopic – as with a sob and staring eyes he turns his face stiffly to the wall.

Like the old woman sent to the Old Aged 'Home', or a retarded child hidden away in an institution, or the man told he has HIV – the antibody of death – floating in his bloodstream, the patient's name soon fades and dies away under the magical curse of a diagnostic word. To the rest of society he slowly becomes the undead, the half-forgotten inhabitant of a limbo land, the Land of Nocebo, the one that lies just beyond the horizons of life.

But in the meantime, back in the bedroom, it is already the following night. Carefully the apocryphal woman has swallowed down her tranquillizer capsule with a glass of water, this time with the green end first.

Carried downwards by the waves of peristalsis, and the wash of water, the capsule meanders from side to side like a confused submarine, voyaging down the long oesophagus towards the stomach. But along with that capsule the woman has swallowed something else: its colour, its texture and emblematic shape, and the mystical name printed upon the packet. And with all of these she has also swallowed the makers and marketers of the capsule, smiling at her from their clean white laboratories. And she has also gulped down the healing charisma of the doctor, the grave glance of his face as he bends over the cluttered desk writing the prescription, and the kindly curl of his mouth as he raises his silvered head and hands it over to her. And along with him are swallowed also all the rituals and symbolic powers of Medical Science, encoded in the talismans of the doctor's office, from the circle of diplomas on his wall to the glitter of his arcane instruments.

Now all of this concoction of symbols and certainties, gulped down with a mouthful of water, begins to seep slowly out of her stomach and into her psyche. Though the capsule has not yet reached the intestine, its site of absorption, the fingers of a soft languor are already beginning to relax the tension of her muscles, loosening the tight knots in her terrified brain.

Meanwhile, deep down in her stomach, the peristaltic waves turn the capsule round and around, so that now it shoots down into the small intestine, black end first. But the woman is unaware of this. For already she is fast asleep, dreaming of a wide calm field, emerald as an aquarium, and of the green bushes and shrubs that have begun to sprout all around her, out of the black, shiny gelatin earth.

CHAPTER 5

✧

The Premenstrual Werewolf

On the 19th November 1981, under the headline 'HARLEY ST ALERT ON PMT WOMEN: **GP's are warned: Treat "animal" syndrome seriously**,' a newspaper for general practitioners called *Doctor* reports on the case of a 29-year-old barmaid, found guilty of threatening with a penknife to kill a policeman. The barmaid is already on probation for manslaughter. Now she is found guilty of this new charge, but surprisingly is not sent to jail. Her defence is that when the incident happened, she was suffering from Premenstrual Tension (or PMT). A famous gynaecologist supports her defence. For two years she has studied inmates at the Holloway women's prison. Many of them, too, had committed their crimes during their PMT, a time of temporary 'loss of control', when the level of the hormone progesterone is low in their bloodstreams. The barmaid should also have had her daily dose of progesterone prescribed by her doctor, but due to an administrative error she never received it. It is the only effective treatment for her condition, she says, and for the disruptive symptoms of Premenstrual Tension. The judge agrees. Without that hormone, the accused woman had revealed 'the hidden animal within her', and so turned to violence and aggression. 'She badly wants to be good,' he concludes as he sets her free, and could not be blamed for her crimes.

★

At the same time (or perhaps it is years later, or even earlier), a man standing at the window watches as the full moon rises slowly over the rooftops. He feels the prickly rash spreading slowly over his skin. Sadly he puts down the newspaper, and the glass of wine. Already it is too late to do anything about it. For now the little pink bumps are beginning to appear all over his body, each one the soil of a sprouting hair follicle. He feels the familiar ache in his jaw, as his teeth begin to elongate and the acidic saliva drips and drips down onto the carpet. With a sigh he looks down at his furry hands and their sharpening claws. Slowly he scratches at the thick bristles growing along his snout. In the moonlight, his eyes are turning an amber yellow, a faint glow in the gathering dusk.

As he climbs through the window, to lope once again across the rooftops, he catches sight of himself in a mirror hung on the wall. For a moment he snarls in bewilderment. Who is that tall, hairy, enraged creature staring back at him from across the room? It is a question that will torture him, that his nightmares will ask of one another again and again, every night until the next new moon. For each time he is left with that same puzzled amnesia, with migraines and blurred eyeballs, with dark stains on his fingertips and curious scratches all over his body, and with a bitter, decaying taste that will linger in his mouth for many days afterwards.

The creature in that mirror is neither animal nor man, fish nor fowl. He is that marginal, mysterious being who in so many places bays at the boundary between animals and men. He is the *lycanthropos*, the man-wolf, the snarling werewolf of our cinematic nightmares.

Of course this furry creature of the night, with his long fangs and hair, has never heard of the premenstrual barmaid or of her lack of progesterone, and yet there are curious connections between them – or rather between the images that they both invoke in our modern iconography.

★

The werewolf, like the lumbering monster of Dr Frankenstein, is part of the cinematic folklore of our age, star of a whole genre of popular horror films. But this modern werewolf of the screen has a much older genealogy. In many ancient mythologies he was believed to be the man who became a wolf by night, but returned by day to human form. In those dark hours of in-between, he was transformed into a wild creature who roamed across moonlit landscapes in search of prey, who ravaged and devoured sleeping people, and animals, and even corpses.

Some of these fated men, the cinema tells us, can turn into wolves at will, others only under the luminous influence of a full moon. Such a man can first become a wolf-man in many ways: sometimes by birth into a blighted heredity, or by spells or curses, or by the contagious bite of a passing werewolf. Once infected, he will be tainted forever, carrying the hairy violence within his blood, a perpetual slave to the cycles of the moon.

In Europe, the werewolf is the scion of Teutonic mythology, and its origins lie deep in southern Scandinavia, and in the wide plains of northern Germany, between the Vistula and the Rhine. Here there was an ancient belief that the souls of living people could leave their bodies, and lead a separate, independent existence. Each person thus had a second self – the Scandinavians called it the *fylgja*, 'the follower' – which could move, act, speak, and exercise its bodily functions just like a human being. Sometimes this second self would appear in human form, sometimes in the form of an animal. Any damage to either of these selves would be felt by the other; and if one died, so did the other. From this fertile northern soil grew the legends of the werewolf – the man who had the power to turn himself into a wolf, in order to attack other men, or to ravage their flocks.

There is an old Norse story of how Sigmund and Sinfjöth accidentally became werewolves, when they dressed themselves in the discarded pelts of two wolves that they found in a forest. Once these skins were on their backs, it was impossible to remove them, or to escape from their powerful contagion. Soon both men began to rage and snarl, and howl like wolves, attacking other people, and biting at one another. On the tenth day of their torment, the wolfskins fell suddenly from their shoulders. Quickly they burnt the furry pelts, till nothing remained, and once again were free from the curse of the werewolf.

These northern, Teutonic werewolves, such as the *werwolf* of Germany and the *varulf* of Norway, have their lupine cousins all over the continent of Europe – from the *volkolak* of Russia, down to the Greek *brukolakas* and the *loup-gaou* of France. Many of the members of this extended family of wolfmen were believed to undergo their violent change every month by the full moonlight, in a cyclical death and rebirth of both their human and their animal selves.

In the version of the myth made popular in horror films, lycanthropy – the transformation of man into wolf – is usually portrayed as a cyclical condition, influenced by the full moon. In that most famous werewolf film of all, *The Wolf Man* of 1941, the young Lawrence Talbot (played by Lon Chaney Jnr), the son of a squire, returns home to Wales after years in America. One full moon, among the woods of Llanwelly, he comes upon a girl being attacked by a werewolf. In the struggle to rescue her, he is bitten by the wolf – who is really the lupine incarnation of Bella, the gipsy – and so becomes a werewolf. From now on, young Talbot cannot escape his terrible fate. He will become a wolf, 'a thing of hair and claws . . . when the wolfbane blooms, and the autumn moon is bright.' He is destined to kill and kill again, until finally he is slain by his own father with the aid of a silver cane.

Most of the early werewolves of Hammer Films or Hollywood were still servants to this traditional full moon. But in other cinematic versions of ancient myth, therianthropy – the metamorphosis of humans into animals – is often the work of men (usually of mad scientists), and not of the moon. As the horrors of the twentieth century have accumulated, many of the films portray how the rays, potions, drugs and 'glandular extracts' of a corrupt science now transform one species into another, turning men into apes, alligators, flies and wolves. In the classic horror film, *The Mad Monster*, made in 1941, the mad Dr Cameron injects the hapless Pedro, his handyman, with an infusion 'brewed from the blood of a wolf'. Soon Pedro is transformed into a werewolf, all hair and fangs, and ready to kill. In a sinister echo of events in Europe, Cameron plans to create an entire army of these wolf-men, that will be invincible in battle. But horror films rarely let such hubris go unpunished. Pedro's first victim is an innocent young girl, but his second is Dr Cameron himself, strangled by the claws of his wolf-man in a lurid climactic scene, just as lightning strikes his laboratory and the fire cremates them both.

Parallel to the werewolf films, there is another tradition of horror movies – one in which women are the ones transformed, often by curses or chemicals, into a variety of animals, such as cats, leopards, cheetahs or panthers. The classic example of the genre – a parable of sexual jealousy and revenge – is *Cat Girl*, made in Britain in 1957. It is the story of Nora, a repressed middle-class English girl, whose husband has an affair with her closest friend, shortly after their marriage. Under the influence of an inherited family curse, and powered by her repressed rage and frustration, Nora becomes 'Leonora', transformed into a deadly cheetah that savages both husband and treacherous friend, as they make love among the trees.

Both horror films and history are usually the tales of one-way transformations. Whether by the lunar powers of nature, or by the lunatic powers of science, it is almost always the human who is turned into the beast, and not the other way round. But what of the reverse direction? While the transformation of a premenstrual barmaid from a monthly 'animal' back into a human needs (according to a certain judge) only a special hormone made by science, that most difficult of permanent transformations – that of a wild animal into a contented man – seems to require (at least on celluloid) only the love of a woman, the pure love of the maiden in *Beauty and the Beast*, turning the man-animal forever into a handsome Prince.

The mythic man-wolf of Europe, loping across the cinema screens, is the furry descendant of a long line of zoomorphic spirits and gods. In ancient legends, at the mythological periphery of the known and ordered world, men and women have often twinned themselves with animals, birds, fish or reptiles. In most of the archaic world – in Greece, Rome, Egypt, India, as well as in Africa and the Americas – the hybrid powers of these magical fusions would stride or swoop everywhere through the misty chimerical air. In Greek mythology, among the many hybrid creatures or gods, there was the raunchy man-goat or Satyr and the man-horse Centaur, and the man-bull Minotaur who hid in the labyrinth of Crete, waiting for his victims, and the Gorgon woman with her hissing serpentine hair and her perilous glance that could turn men into stone, and the little mischievous Pan of all the glades and forests, horned and bearded like a goat. And there were the more complex collages too, like the Chimera – a mythical being with a lion's head, a goat's body and the long pointed tail of a dragon – or the hag-faced Harpies with their bears' ears and the feathered bodies of birds. In ancient Egypt there lived the Sphinx, a creature with a human head and the body of a lion, and Horus of Memphis, the falcon-headed god who carried the sun's orb over his head, and Seker, hawk-headed god of the Dead, Sekhmet with the head of a lioness, Sebek with the physiognomy of a crocodile, and Anubis of the black ears and the long pointed jackal snout. In Indian mythology, it is still

Ganesh the popular son of Siva and Parvati, a man-god with the head of an elephant, who is the deity of wisdom, good luck, prudence, and the removal of all obstacles. And even in Europe, the seductive woman-fish or Mermaid still lures us into the salt-water depths of the mind, in counterpoint to that wily and ubiquitous landsman, Old Nick the Devil, with his cloven-hoofs and horns, his forked tail and cold, mesmeric eyes.

In Ancient Greece, myths about wolves and gods were common, for it was King Lycaon, son of Pelagos, whom Zeus turned from man into wolf, and who was worshipped in a wolf-temple, or Lyceum. In Arcadia, a region of Greece plagued by wolves, a cult flourished of the Wolf-Zeus, with an annual gathering held on Mount Lycaeus. Here the priests would brew a sacrificial feast, a mixture of meat and human parts. One mouthful of this hideous brew and you became a wolf yourself, unable to return to human form unless, for a period of nine years, you never ate of human flesh again. In Rome too, it was well known that some men could transform themselves into a wolf – the long-fanged *versi-pellis*, or turn-pelt – a creature that could ravage both sheep and sleeping humans.

Some belief in werewolves, or in other were-animals, is found almost everywhere. It is found in warm countries and in chilly ones, as often among the snow blizzards of Scandinavia as in the tropical rain-forests of the Congo basin. Everywhere in this universal myth, a human takes the form of a beast of prey, usually the predatory animal of that region. In Europe it is mostly the wolf and the bear. In India, China, Japan, and the rest of Asia, it is the tiger; in most of Africa, the leopard or the lowly hyena.

In North Africa, the Berbers of Morocco still believe in *boudas*, men who can turn into hyenas at nightfall, and resume human shape in the morning; while further south, among the Banyang people of West Cameroon, all people are believed to have *babu*, or were-animals, animal-doubles that are the spirit extensions of the self. Like the *fylgja* of the Teutons, these mystical and malevolent animals live and act in an independent way, in a parallel world alongside our own. At night they may leave the body of their sleeping owner and roam silently among the villages, causing illness, misfortune or death to other people. Like the werewolves of Europe, any injury to these animal-selves of the night will show itself next day, when they revert to human form. Sores and scratches on the body in the morning are seen as the mystical marks of such a were-animal's wanderings, while an attack of whooping cough is seen as the pantings of a leopard-self, one that had been chased by hunters the night before.

In European witchcraft of the sixteenth and seventeenth centuries, some women were also believed to turn themselves into animals or imps, or to copulate fiercely with invisible demons. These women often had 'familiars', either small animals or their own animal-doubles, that they sent to bring fear or disaster to members of the community. 'There came to her a thynge like a black dog,' reads the testimony of a young girl, in an Essex witch trial of 1566, 'with a face like an ape, a short taile, a cheine and sylver whystle (to her thinking) about his neck, and a payre of horns on his head, and brought in his mouth the key of the milkhouse door.' This hybrid 'thynge' was a phantom, demonic animal that had been sent to demand butter from her by the witch Agnes Waterhouse, a woman whose tell-tale 'diverse spottes in her face' later doomed her to death on the charge of witchcraft.

An old witch's spell of transformation into one of these animal doubles or *doppelgängers* – a 'witch-hare' – still survives, in all its poignancy:

> I shall go into a hare,
> With sorrow and such,

And mickle care.
And I shall go in the Devil's name,
Aye, 'till I come home again.

The salient sign of the modern werewolf, and the technical delight of make-up artists, is the hair that suddenly sprouts from its body and face. In other traditions too, there is no shortage of such hairy and mythical beings. In the Babylonian epic of the hero Gilgamesh ('his two-thirds was a god, his one-third a man'), Enkidu, his friend and former enemy, is described as the 'wild or natural man' who grew up among the wild beasts of the desert. His body was covered with coarse, matted hair just like that of Samuquan's, the god of cattle. On his head the hair was like a woman's, 'growing like the harvest', and it waved in the breeze like the hair of Nisoba, the goddess of corn. Enkidu was a being who was 'innocent of mankind', a part of nature rather than society, one who 'knew nothing of the cultivated land'.

Huge, hairy and wild – modern Enkidus still live on in the depths of those blurred photographs, or in the hollows of their invisible footprints on the slopes of the Himalayas. The Yeti, the Sasquatch and the Wild Man are still pacing, naked and wary, at the very periphery of the human world. These mythical creatures are the logical descendants of ancient Trolls and Giants, of Enkidu and Esau, and of all our hirsute and shadowy cousins who once swung from the distant branches of the family tree.

Such hairy men at the edges of society are wild, and like the werewolf, often considered dangerous. In southern Africa, there lives still the *Utokoloshe* of Zulu mythology, and the *Uthikoloshe* of the Xhosas – evil spirits that appear to humans in the form of small, gnarled, hairy homunculi, who live near deep waters, as deep as their sexual appetites. They are the tricksters who lead you astray, who tempt you into confusion or crime. To look them in the face is death.

★

The werewolf is the hairy man of myth, but why in particular *hair*? The answer to that riddle lies in the symbolic significance of hair in so many human societies.

Anthropologists have long noted the curious and emblematic quality of hair, and how everywhere it is seen as if it were a vital, renewable crop, one that sprouts from birth out of our fertile scalps. In all cultures it is the marker of sexual maturity, an emblem of puberty and fertility. From the tentative, whispy moustache or beard, to the secret flowering of the pubic garden, it is the visible sign of an adult status. It always has a sexual significance too, as if it were semen gushing from the top of a phallic head, a sign of both potency and youth. Without this sperm-hair there is only castration and decay, as poor Samson realized, but much too late, as he stood eyeless in Gaza, among the reverberating echoes of Delilah's scissors.

Hair of the scalp and face is also a type of blank slate on which people write messages to one another, telling who is what in society, and where, and why. The trim and arrangement of our hair – how it is cut, shaped, and gathered together – are all strands in the complex network of shared meanings that link us together, for they are signals of gender and age, ritual power or social status. Hair is an important part of the social radar of our lives, a vibrant but silent language between us.

Priests and officiants from many faiths have always used this language of hair to signal their symbolic power, or special holiness. Greek clerics and rabbis today, sadhus and ayatollahs, still display their ritual status and role by the dogmatic cut of their hair, moustache and beard. Contrasted with these long-haired holy men, and living far out of sight in that sealed building high on the hill, the cropped scalp of the Buddhist monk, the military recruit, the collaborator or the convict all show their submission to the rules of order, to the lonely yoke of a special type of discipline.

Out on the margins of society, the heads and beards of the

rebel, the hermit, the hippy, and the artist all carry on them a different set of messages – the public signs of a wild disorder, a bacchanalia of the scalp and the mind. Like the Rastafarian with his dreadlocks of the lions of Judah, the style of their hair puts them outside the ordered structures of bourgeois life. Such long, wild, disordered hair in men or in women, wrote the anthropologist C. R. Hallpike in a famous essay, are a public signal of nonconformity, showing to all how they are less subject to social control than the average man.

And that average man stares back askance at all those scalps bursting with wild, ungardened hair. He feels strange, curiously uneasy down to the very roots of his own hair follicles, at all this hairy disorder. Nervously he runs his fingers along the neat furrows of his own, domesticated scalp. Nervously he shudders at all the other anomalous messages that he has received: those from the bearded woman, the bald man, the crew-cut girl, the baby with the hairy pelt. But he nods with respect at the short-cropped hair of the mourner, remembering that ancient cry of the Prophet Jeremiah: 'Cut off thine hair, O Jerusalem, and cast it away, and take up a lamentation in high places.'

In both language and myth, women, hair and the imagery of sex are often closely intertwined. Long and flowing hair can be the signal of individuality or of an unbridled sensuality, but it can also convey other, less obvious messages on the nature of femininity. In the everyday slang of nineteenth-century England, for example, a 'hairy' was a 'hatless slum girl', a 'hairy bit' an 'amorous and attractive wench', and sexual desire 'to feel hairy'. The act of sex was 'to get one's hair cut', the penis was a 'hair-divider', and the vulva a 'hairy oracle', a 'hairy ring', or the mythical county of Hairyfordshire.

While women's long hair is the symbol of their gender (and of sexuality), it can also carry an extra and dangerous message. For in many human cultures, long hair is also the symbol of *animality*, the sign of the beast, the sign of Nature, and of those who live or work among it. Often, like Esau and Enkidu before him, it is the sign of uncouth marginal men, of the fields or the forests or the distant mountains. At these outer fringes of human society, where humanity ends and the wilderness begins, men and animals seem to blur together, their coarse pelts woven into the same ancient, seamless texture. Esau was such a hairy hunter, a rough man of the fields – unlike his brother Jacob the 'smooth man', that 'plain man, dwelling in tents'.

The flowing hair of femaleness thus carries with it the subliminal tinge of Nature, of a life on the margins of ordered society. Hallpike has written how, in the spurious equation of so many cultures, long hair places one outside the male conception of 'human society'. 'Outside society,' he wrote, 'equals hairiness equals animality.'

For centuries some men have seen woman as the 'weaker vessel', inferior both morally and physically to men, and deserving of her subordination. Others saw woman as the evil temptress, a source of pollution, and a danger to man's spirituality. Thus theologians from Christianity, Judaism and Islam have all banned women from the priesthood, and the exercise of religious authority. Underlying much of their misogyny has been the image of women as part of 'Nature' – their bodies, instincts and emotions more subject to the tides and cycles of the natural world than to the rational and ordered world of men. Some early misogynists even argued that woman has no soul – that cardinal sign of humanness. Even as late as 1646, George Fox, founder of the Society of Friends, encountered on his travels some people in Nottingham who confidently assured him that 'women have no soul . . . no more than a goose.'

This idea of women as embedded in Nature, as somehow more primitive, pre-social, or even animal-like than men, has not disappeared along with the decline of religion and myth. Witness Charles Darwin's infamous remark, as he dismissed the 'less highly evolved female brain' as 'characteristic of the lower races, and therefore of a past and lower state of civilization'.

Even today, this image of female 'animality', embedded in the natural world, is reflected in masculine slang for women or their sexuality: Puss, Bird, Vixen, Chick, Cat, Kitten, Cow, Bitch or Hen are the names some men still give to their lovers or wives.

The image of the animal-other – of other human beings (male or female) as being animal, or part-animal – is really the projected image of the *animal-double* – the one we all carry within ourselves. But this double – representing to Jungians man's primitive and instinctual nature – contains a false image of animality, a caricature of a hairy, violent and sexual creature, both cruel and competitive. This bogus idea of what animals are is one that we incorporate into our ideas of self. The 'animal within', the 'lupine urge', and the 'instinctual nature' of man are all parts of this model of the split-self, a self that is both social *and* anti-social, and which contains within it both 'human' and 'animal' characteristics. Above all, the model of the 'animal within' is one of guilty animals and innocent men. In the cinematic myth of the werewolf, the inner guilt of this animal-half becomes visible, as on the screen the creature of hair and fangs climbs out of its human shell – that innocent slave to the swollen moon – and roams through the night once more.

What we call 'animals' can be seen as only the feathered or furry screens onto which we project the fears of our own nature, the dark side of our own psychic moons. They are the victims of our ideas of self, the repository of our sense of sin. To erase the pain of this inner knowledge, we are hunting them to extinction. The holocaust of animals shows this ironic paradox of the hunter's mind – for in a doomed bid to kill the animal within, he must slaughter the animal without.

This perpetual dialectic between the ideas of 'human' and those of 'animal' has taken place both inside and outside the borders of the mind, since the very beginning of human history. The clash between the two is still played out in everyday life, in the mythology of many cultures, in the horror films of the present day, in the literary struggle of Captain Ahab and the whale Moby Dick (symbol of untamed Nature), in the annual pursuit of the fox, deer, quail or duck, and in the careful violence of the Iberian bull-fight – that ritualized combat between the two halves of the Minotaur.

But History tells us – not politely, but with a loud shout in the ear – that this dialectic is the disease of all human life, that our own *human* tale is one of violence, pain, blood almost every month of the year. And that all our wars, conquests and colonization involve at some level the 'animalization' of the enemy, his expulsion from human society, and his conversion into the hairy prey of the hunter. We can see this clearly in his coarse physiognomy on the propaganda posters of war or revolution. There is the shameful hair of the beast that sprouts from his cheeks and chin, the grotesque ears and nostrils, the huge bushy eyebrows that shadow the glare of his yellowish eyes. Yet look more closely, for there is something oddly familiar about that face, though we have never seen it before. As if from a paper mirror, or from a dark cinema screen, it stares back at us with that same enraged, puzzled look. In the background we can see the early rays of the rising moon, and feel the first hair follicles sprouting all over our skin.

In that famous fairy-tale, a young girl – Little Red Riding Hood – is sent to carry cakes to her grandmother, in a cottage hidden in the woods. On the path she meets a Wolf, a hungry predator who tries to lure her away. 'Oh, no, thank you,' says the girl politely, and continues on her journey. The Wolf disappears, but he has really run ahead to get to the cottage

71

before her, while she meanders on among the trees. In the cottage he quickly eats the grandmother, dresses himself in her frilly nightdress, and climbs into her bed to await the girl. Now in the dramatic core of the tale, the door opens and pubescent Beauty and disguised-Beast stare at one another across the room. 'Oh Grandmother, what big teeth you have!' cries the girl in wonder. 'All the better to eat you with, my dear,' replies the Wolf, as he gobbles her down as a delicate dessert. Some while later a hunter (or in some versions, a woodcutter) enters the cottage, to find the Wolf fast asleep and snoring loudly. Realizing what has happened, he takes out his knife and slits open its swollen belly. Grandmother, near the end of her life, and Little Red Riding Hood, near the beginning, are both reborn at the same instant from the moist, hairy belly of the Wolf. The brave hunter, midwife of this double Caesarian birth, and the little girl embrace one another. In the final scene of the tale, all manner of significant symbols are blended together. Carrying her red menstrual cloak, the hymen-hood flung back across her shoulders, Little Red Riding Hood smiles up at her handsome rescuer. In the bed rests Grandmother, on the ground there lies the dying Wolf, his belly pregnant now with rocks and stones.

The child psychologist Bruno Bettelheim has offered his own interpretation of this Wolf motif in fairy-tale and folklore. He sees it as the expression of the girl's struggle with her pubertal problems, with the oedipal conflicts of a budding sexuality, for which she is emotionally unprepared. It shows her ambivalent attitude towards the male, and how he is split into two opposing images: 'the dangerous seducer who, if given into, turns into the destroyer of the grandmother and the girl', and 'the hunter, the responsible, strong, and rescuing father figure'. This conflict between big bad Wolf and Man is that between 'id and ego-superego', between the pleasure principle and the reality principle.

But the Wolf is more than just the male seducer. He also represents all the 'asocial, animalistic tendencies within ourselves', and those same tendencies within the hunter himself. The Wolf, the 'animal within us', is thus a metaphor for our 'propensity for acting violently or irresponsibly to gain our goals'.

In the fairy-tale of Little Red Riding Hood, as in the recent film *The Company of Wolves*, Man and Wolf are split wide apart, in order that one of them may die, so that the other may live. But in the older myth of the werewolf they live on together, fused into the alternating body of a Man-Wolf, as he hunts by moonlight for other grandmothers, in other cottages among the woods.

How did the werewolf legends begin, and why do they return in such cycles to haunt us? The psychiatrist Robert Eisler has explained this by his own, rather unusual theory of evolution, published in 1951. The lycanthrope, he wrote, is only a stage in human development. We are all descended from an 'original peaceful fruit-eating *bon sauvage* of the primeval virginal forest'. In those far-off days we were 'a peaceful, frugivorous, non-fighting and not even jealous animal'. But our Edenic life was ended forever by famine, and by the forced mutation of behaviour that resulted: above all, by the imitation of the ways of animal predators. To Eisler, 'civilization' really begins with the wearing of clothes – at first the pelt of a dead wolf – and then by the imitation of the wolf's behaviour. The children of the fruit-eaters then become the new packs of carnivorous hunters. Even now, he writes, we are all descended from those ancient 'males of the carnivorous lycanthropic variety', and still carry within ourselves folk memories of those bloody and distant days. Among all the bustle of modernity, and behind the façades of civilization, we are still at the mercy of that 'archetypal lupine urge'.

Clip-clopping along the sidewalks of the modern city on

73

her high stiletto heels, there still walks, according to Eisler, another of those lupine throwbacks. Striding among the sky-scrapers and the flicker of traffic lights, with bloodied lips and fingernails, or drawing her long smooth nyloned legs up into cabs and chauffeured cars, is the creature he called the 'Lady in the Fur'.

She is the female double of the Wolf or Don Juan, an urban carnivore and man-eater, wearing – even on a hot summer's day – the skins of slaughtered animals: mink, leopard, sable or fox. With her fur pelt and needle-pointed nails, he writes, it's as if she 'had just indulged in an omophagic orgy of tearing live animals to pieces'. In her talons and fur, she is a beast of prey, one to be stalked only by a 'big dame hunter'.

Other modern lycanthropes, says Eisler, are the sadist or the war-monger, and both are throwbacks to that earlier behaviour pattern, emerging from 'the abyss of the collective unconscious'. For the sake of the future, he says, our only hope is to throw off 'the fatal wolf's mask', and tame the 'archetypal' beast' within ourselves.

This vision of vegetarian lads and lasses gently picking fruit amongst the fragrant trees is redolent of the Arcadian fantasies of Watteau and Fragonard. It seems part of Eisler's nostalgia for a pre-war or pre-industrial Garden of Eden, for a world of innocence and settled order before 1939, when the wild bayings of the wolf-packs began. But it is a world that has gone forever. For the werewolves continue to live on among us, waiting patiently for a cloudless moon.

Today the werewolf, and all the other hairy man-animals, have been exiled to the outer margins of the mind, to the Himalayas of our imagination. Rarely do they climb down off the cinema screen, and into our daily lives. Those that do are quickly confined to the white-coated wards of psychiatric hospitals. But it was not always thus. In the Middle Ages and after, such beings – real or imagined – were often burnt alive as being possessed by the Devil. There is the legendary

case of Peter Stubb, the German werewolf, who was believed
to turn himself into a wolf with the aid of a 'magic girdle',
a gift to him from the Devil. For twenty-five years he murdered and mutilated women, children and livestock, until
his capture and execution in the year 1590. Between 1520 and
1630, there were 30,000 other such werewolves recorded in
Europe, and on the cinema screen the hairy plague continues
to this very day.

These days such hybrid man-animals are usually considered to be walking specimens of a new disease – *lycanthropy*
– 'the belief that one has been transformed into an animal,
or behaviour suggestive of such a belief'. Such is its power
that, in a few rare cases, it can manifest as cannibalism, sadism or even necrophilia.

In 1988, in the journal *Psychological Medicine*, a group of
psychiatrists told of their own, rather milder cases of lycanthropy at the McLean Hospital in Boston. Their clinical narratives include two Cats, two Wolves, a Dog, a Gerbil, a
Bird, a Rabbit, a Bengal Tiger and two ill-defined 'Unspecifieds'. The behaviour of these patients is reported by the
doctors as bizarre, psychotic, and most zoological. The two
Wolves and the Dog howl at one another in the ward,
the Bengal Tiger growls, the Gerbil sleeps under his hospital
bed and twitches, the Rabbit hops about, the Bird chirps
and flaps his arms, while the 'Unspecifieds' crawl around,
hooting and howling, and stamp their feet or defecate in
the rooms.

They tell in some detail the story of the unfortunate
'Patient 8', a 24-year-old depressed man who for thirteen
years has believed that he is a cat, trapped inside the body of
a human. He has known this ever since the secret was im-
parted to him by the family cat, that same animal who later
taught him 'cat language'. Though employed, he continued
to spend most of his spare time in feline activities. He lived
with cats, had sexual intercourse with them, hunted with
them, and frequented cat night spots in preference to their

human equivalents. 'His greatest – but unrequited – love', they write, 'was for a tigress in a local zoo. He hoped one day to release her.'

Their tale concludes with a sombre summary of his unsuccessful treatment, for his 'lycanthropic delusions' were not cured. Against all the evidence, he clung firm to his cat beliefs, even after medication with haloperidol, antidepressants and carbamazepine, and six years of 'insight-orientated psychotherapy'.

There is something poignant, but also emblematic about poor 'Patient 8'. He seems to be a clear symbol of something, but of what? As we listen to the mewings from his white-tiled menagerie, we realize that we, too, could be the 'unspecified' in someone else's case-history. Often enough we are the semi-beasts in another's bestiary, someone seen across the table or the town, or across the borders of war.

Poor lonely and deluded 'Patient 8'. Yet in some way he points the way to an image of liberation, of a counter-life of the soul, a failed leap to freedom, a wild roam across the rooftops from mortgages into madness. In some unconscious way he inverts the delusion of progress, travels backwards along the tracks of linear time. In his madness he is the sad architect of a reverse evolution, of the transformation of man back into animal.

Whether lycanthropy is madness or metaphor, the modern cinematic myth of the werewolf is the descendant of ancient folk theories that were once used to explain human cruelty, insanity and the recurring turmoil of war.

In the models of Premenstrual Tension, created by males and by medical science, women are seen as the slaves of a cyclical moon, as violent and irrepressible when 'the hidden animal within her' emerges in its monthly rage, with fangs and flying hair, and spills its contagious blood across the ordered certainties of masculine life.

In a very similar way, the body of the mythic werewolf is

also transformed, every month of the lunar year, with sudden wild outbreaks of hair, that cultural mark of 'animality' – and of 'femaleness' – followed by pain, chaos, and the spilling of blood. Thus the werewolf myths carry with them the feeling of *déjà vu*, for it is the *female* cycle of the menses that is being imitated here, but in a distorted form, and blended with an overlay of pure male violence. Like the 'couvade' – those psychosomatic symptoms of stomach cramps and nausea that some men have when their wives give birth – this myth can be seen as an imitation of female life, as an exaggerated but envious mimicry of their bodily cycles and fertility.

'The body is a natural symbol supplying some of our richest sources of metaphor,' wrote the anthropologist Mary Douglas. From the forms and feelings of the body we learn a vocabulary of metaphors for understanding our daily lives – from 'left' wing to 'right' wing, from the 'head' of a government, to the 'heart' of a community. In the myth of the werewolf, it is a caricatured version of the female menstrual cycle that provides men with a model or metaphor for understanding their own history, and the contagious, cyclical violence of their own lives. The wars, cruelty, massacres and murders carried out by men are seen in these myths as recurrent outbreaks of hairy 'animality'. Thus the story of the werewolf – a man whose violence is slave to the cyclical forces of nature, outside his control – can be seen as an image of *male* menstruation, and of the many tensions that precede it.

Hair, Moon and Blood form an awesome trinity of powerful female symbols at the very core of the werewolf myth – a myth about the violence of men. Together they blend the grand cycles of the cosmos, and the repetitive violence of male life, with the terrors of contagion and of the animal-self.

The wolf-man may lack the Brylcreemed charm of his screen cousin Dracula, but he is just as contagious. Just as there is sensual awakening in the kiss of Count Dracula – a sort of sexual rabies from his love-bite – so can lycanthropy be transmitted by the bite of a werewolf.

This image of the contagion of evil resonates with some of the modern folk imagery of AIDS, in both popular discourse and the media. The fatal and invisible HIV virus evokes an infectious terror in many who hear of it, along with a fear of its victims, and of contamination by the blood, spittle and sperm that leak from their bodies. The images of AIDS in modern life are those of an invisible, immoral contagion, one carried among us by marginal people in their life-styles or body-fluids – not hairy and mythical wolf-men this time, but homosexuals, drug addicts, prostitutes or immigrants. Above all, the fear of AIDS – like the more ancient fear of the bite of a werewolf – is a fear of the contagion of moral chaos, of the ordered world turned upside-down, and of a spreading epidemic of 'animal' sexuality.

The contagious blood and saliva of the werewolf are also the mythic, male parallels of menstrual blood. In many religions and cultures, men have always had a terror of this blood's pollution, and of its power to weaken their virility, blight crops or ruin the food. 'There is nothing so unclean as a woman in her period,' wrote Father Jerome in the fourth century, while three centuries later Bishop Isidore of Seville insisted that the very touch of a menstruating woman could prevent fruit from ripening, or cause plants to die. Menstruating women, say the English 'old wives' tales', should never enter a dairy or the butter won't churn, the cream won't rise, and the cheese won't set. During their periods, all such women were dangerous: they should be kept away not only from men, but from sacred places, and from the preparation of meals. But the woman herself was also in danger, prone to illness if she should swim, wash her hair, or even bathe her feet in cold water. Even today, some tribes in Africa and the Pacific confine young women each month to a 'menstrual hut' at the very periphery of the village, protecting them from danger, and the men from the dangerous powers of their menstrual blood.

In modern society, some of this male fear of the polluting power of menstrual blood seems to be controlled by the metronomic, twenty-eight-day beat of the contraceptive pill, as it rigidly binds the woman's cycles to the clock time of the industrial calendar. Today the pill makes menstruation a phenomenon which is safe for men, tamed and predictable, something easily counted and calculated in advance. In doing so it also divides women's bodies from one another, breaking down the synchronized menstruation of those who live together.

Parallel with this fear of menstrual blood is often another ancient belief – in the power of the Full Moon over 'lunatics', animals, and especially women. In many arcane traditions and mythologies, the Moon itself is seen as female, and the Sun as male. The medieval alchemist Hermes Trismegistus wrote of The One, the central principle of all life: 'The Sun is its father and the Moon its Mother. The Wind has carried it in its belly, and the Earth is its nurse.' In these myths, the lunar cycle of the menses links women's physiology to the greater cycles of the cosmic bodies. In mythological terms, it is an image of women controlled by nature. But there is always another side to this idea – for these monthly menses also place women outside the power of males, making them subject instead to mysterious cosmic or hormonal forces.

In the myth of the werewolf, men too are subject to the whims of the Moon, that great cosmic puppeteer. As the moon controls the menses, so does it control the violence of the man-wolf, the animal incarnation of man, in both cinema and myth. The power of the moon is the plea of mitigation of the werewolf. In every generation such violent men will return scarred from their outbreaks of rage and of war, their cyclical wanderings beyond the borders of human society. Like the premenstrual barmaid before them, they will plead with the judges of History, quoting the legend of the were-wolf – 'It was not your fault,' the judge will say, 'you badly want to be good.' 'Yes, it was the Moon that made me do it,' the man-wolf will reply, 'or the Sun or my Stars – or the hidden animal-within, the one driven by those invisible rays, leaking from the cosmos.'

Now at last it is time to return to the werewolf, as it turns slowly back into man in the rising dawn. As he falls exhausted onto the blood-stained sheets, at the end of that muddy trail of hair and paw-prints across the carpet, the man can feel the first throbs of the nightmare screaming inside his skull. It is a confused, Technicolor vision of forests and fields, of a wild lope across a luminous landscape, of the stares of the villagers, and of his blurred reflection in the waters of a moonlit pond.

And through the window, we in the audience can see how slowly in the night sky, and in the bedroom itself, the Full Moon is sinking below the horizon. We watch as it draws its blue and shadowy veil behind it across the stars. Now the Moon has gone, and it continues to glow only on the dark side of our minds. And surely we know that it will reappear one day, and again and yet again, to drag from their sleep the madman, the dreamer, and that werewolf of war.

CHAPTER 6

✧

The Medusa Machine

I am sitting in the doctors' room of the medical centre, chewing on a sesame-seed bun, when the telephone rings and a woman screams so violently into my ear that a shower of seeds scatters across the carpet. 'He's gone!' she shouts. 'He's gone! Oh my God, he's gone! And he's on the floor!' The bun will have to wait. I run downstairs towards the car-park, quickly pulling his medical notes out of the filing cabinet on the way. I am newly qualified, still worried and fresh amongst the daily dramas of medical practice. The man on the floor is ninety-two years old.

With my foot flat on the accelerator, the black bag on the seat beside me, the little car leaps through the streets, jumping over traffic lights and crossings in a wild gymkhana of horns and flashing headlights.

I arrive at the house in the tiny cul-de-sac, and jump out, sprinting across the street and into the opened door. It is a noisy summer afternoon in mid-June, with the roar of cars and trucks in the hot air, the Boeings flying overhead to Heathrow airport, the treetops full of the shrill gossip of a thousand birds.

A middle-aged woman sits sobbing in the dark hallway, at the bottom of a flight of stairs. She is pointing at a closed door on the right. With a nod to her I put my hand on the doorknob, my mind flicking its fingers busily through the pages of a medical textbook. But the door is either locked, or held against me. I push harder with one hand, and then with the other, and then grip it tightly with both. The door gives just a bit, but then slams shut again. Someone inside – or perhaps some*thing* – is pushing it back against me. I look down at the woman on the stairs for help, but she has begun to moan and sway, shaking her head into a large crumpled handkerchief.

Outside in the street, the birds in the trees seem to have fallen silent. But here in the hallway, from inside the closed room on the other side of the door, there is a sudden commotion. It sounds like a crowd of people, an excited mob yelling to one another in a shriek of crisis. I see a febrile, grasping, caring crowd, gathered around the old man and trying to resuscitate him. Are they neighbours or friends? Are they mouth-to-mouth men, or chest-pumping women?

I try the door again, and then step back in a bewildered recoil. For the crowd have begun to laugh, a tidal wave of chuckles and giggles that rolls round the room, splashing its spray across my face.

Among all this hilarity, the woman sobs on. In my mind, I leap frantically on to the next chapter of the textbook, and then to the next, but the pages of the book are blank and unhelpful.

Now the crowd are shouting again, and among them I hear a high squeaky hermaphrodite voice, and then laughter again.

Mentally I close the textbook. I put down my bag, and pull on my medical face. Like a rugby player, I throw my full weight and shoulders hard against the door, and then suddenly it opens – but only a bit – so that I can peer in, periscoping my neck around its edge.

Inside, the room is empty – the giggling crowd has slipped away – or rather, not completely empty. On the floor lies a pale form, an imperfect alabaster statue of an old man slumped right against the door. I notice something hollow and empty about his mouth, for his dentures have fallen out of it and rolled across the floor. Now they are lying on their side, smiling up at the flickering, laughing screen of a television set. It is tuned into a comedy programme, a 'situation comedy', but what that situation is remains unclear. Within the machine the voices cackle and talk, the high voice tells a joke again, and then laughs. But the picture on the screen is blurred, fragmented into an abstract kaleidoscope of lights and colours, pulsing and shimmering like an animated painting by Jackson Pollock or Klee.

Looking down at the scene, I realize that all the colour, laughter and talk of a ninety-two-year-old life has somehow been vacuumed out of him, sucked into the machine, and then scattered across its screen.

Cold and silent, as if frozen by the gaze of a Medusa, the old man lies like a forgotten doll, or a perfectly carved automaton, slumped on the shelf of a toy museum.

For centuries we have delighted in the creation of automata, in making moving and mechanical models of men, animals or birds. It is a craft which reached its peak in Europe in the eighteenth century, during the birth pangs of the Industrial Revolution. Hundreds of automata were produced at that time in the northern part of the continent, especially in Switzerland, France and Germany. The philosopher Jean-Jacques Rousseau of Geneva, son of a watchmaker, was the one who first coined the word *automaton* to describe men or women appearing to be machines, but later the meaning was reversed, and the word often came to mean an anthropomorphic machine. The earliest automata were beautiful musical clocks, crafted of wood and metal, with tiny gears and springs inside them, while on the outside there were finely carved displays of moving figures or twittering birds. Among the eighteenth-century creators of these new wonders was the Frenchman Jacques de Vaucanson who built a famous three-dimensional duck that, to the amazement of spectators, appeared to drink, eat and digest food, and even to cackle and swim. On the human side, he made an artificial flautist who could play twelve different tunes on his little flute, a mechanical mandolin player, and a girl who could tap rhythmically on a tiny tambourine.

The Swiss engineer Pierre Jacquet-Droz and his son Henri-Louis were other grand-masters of the automaton art. So lifelike were some of their creations that on one occasion both men were arrested by bewildered officials, and accused of the crime of sorcery. Many of their creations are still to be seen in the museum at Neuchâtel in Switzerland, that same one visited by Mary Shelley, mother of Frankenstein, in the year 1816. Their masterpiece was a life-sized boy, created in 1774, who sat at a desk dressed in velvet and lace. He was capable of writing almost any message on a piece of paper – provided it was less than forty characters long – with a pen held tightly in his pudgy little hand. They also built another mechanical boy, an artist who could draw four different sketches, and a famous female automaton – a young lady dressed in the latest Swiss style, who played with tiny carved fingers on a miniature clavichord, rhythmically swaying and bending with the music.

It was an era of famous fakes too, like the notorious Chess Player, a turbaned Turk with a long pipe and a curly moustache, built by the Baron Wolfgang von Kempelen in 1769. For years this was exhibited in different parts of Europe, and was seen and admired by thousands – among them many famous writers and scientists – but it was a fake all the same. The soul of the machine was a dwarf, a tiny man who crouched within the bowels of its bogus machinery, pulling silently at its hidden levers.

This taste for automata declined later in the nineteenth century, when mass-produced moving toys and dolls began to appear. Among their producers was Thomas Edison, inventor of the light bulb, who made phonographs tiny enough to fit inside a crying doll, making up to five hundred a day in his factory in New Jersey. These toys were the ancestors of the little beeping battery-driven robots and androids of today – the ones that jerk their way, lights flashing, across our carpets and floors, with tiny microchips inside them instead of dwarfs.

By the end of the last century, under the stern metronomic eye of the factory clock, almost all of industrial society had become a sort of grand automaton. As in Fritz Lang's cinematic parable *Metropolis*, made in 1926, workers were now the regimented cogs, gears, and soft moving parts of the meta-machine of modern life. The new industrial city itself, its human and clockwork gears meshed together, began to sprawl and spread across the landscapes of Europe and North America, glittering and throbbing like a giant machine.

Today countless anthropomorphic robots and automata whirr away against the noisy backdrops of industrial society. Machines are everywhere. We live among the pulse of their little cold hearts, the grinding of their metal organs, the inscrutable stare of their luminous consoles.

But machines are no longer just curiosities, or toys. In industry they have become the iron masters of the production-line, harsh tyrants with quick minds of silicon or wire. Other machines are like secretaries that can type, talk or make calculations; translate languages, argue or take messages. Some can play chess, keep the time, direct traffic or hurl missiles at one another. Swift machines can fly us around the world, skimming over the surface of the sea or deep underneath it, or zoom far and free into space to circle the globe. They can dig holes in the ground, in cities and towns, heat houses or cool fridges, carry coal, build ports and railroads – and then demolish them.

The machine is the new Hermes of the information age, a whispering messenger throwing our words or pictures around the world, bouncing them off satellites, faxing them instantly from continent to continent in an interconnecting network of electronic synapses.

With a small black one-eyed machine, we can turn each

other into temporary statues, freeze a gesture or a glance, and then quickly transform it into a piece of celluloid. Everywhere we look we can see these temporary, paired statues – photographer and subject – posing like painted manikins against a landscape, the one smiling at the machine, the other one frowning into it. Year after photographic year we ourselves become more like photographs, as multiples of pale negatives are printed on our flesh, the xerox copies of an identical self.

The streets and highways of the world are now filled with that most ubiquitous machine of all – the motor car. It has become the individualized carapace of the personality, a hollow scuttling scarab painted in the livery of our inner dreams. In the daily rush hours of modern life, it seems to metamorphose instantly into a fish, a metal salmon with glassy eyes and a silver fin, leaping in and out of the asphalt rivers of the city, as it swims its way swiftly upstream towards its breeding grounds in the suburbs.

These millions of machines – as they creep into our lives, and flaunt their mimicry of our abilities – have become the new cousins of our extended family, our cynical relatives of plastic and steel. We have created them to serve us, but like all the Frankensteins and Golems before them, they are indifferent to our human concerns.

The old man, alone in his room with a television set, is at the mercy of a modern descendant of the Medusa, that monster of ancient Greek myth, and of her two sisters, Stheno and Euryale – all three with wild boar tusks on their faces, bronzed hands, golden wings, and complex hairdos of writhing serpents. To look any of them in the face was death, a metamorphosis into a statue of stone – or even into a mute machine.

Every night he sits in his furnished cube, and stares intently with an increasingly un-furnished face into her square cyclopic eye. His body is already part-machine, with a steel hip joint, a plastic artery, an electronic ear, and a battery-driven pacemaker implanted deep within his heart.

Now, as he stares at that hard Medusa face, the rays of her long hair hissing and slithering in the indoor breeze, he realizes that he himself is slowly becoming an automaton, a life-sized model of an old man, sculpted in a chilly white stone. And he knows also that someone, somewhere is slowly switching him off, unplugging and disconnecting him, inch by cold inch, as the warm summer days roll on.

Suddenly he is at the birth of a great realization. For the first time he understands one of the central riddles of his life. Excitedly he gets to his feet, to tell everyone what he has just understood. He opens his mouth, he begins to speak, but at that very instant the crowd bursts out laughing at him – and then his heart stops dead, and the newly born smile rolls out of his mouth, and onto the floor.

Surrounded by our new synthetic kin, we have learnt new ways of seeing ourselves. The machines of daily life provide us with a repertoire of metaphors, lenses through which we perceive the structure and functions of our own human bodies. The pipes of sanitation, the electrical gadgetry within the home, the computer, the tape-recorder and the internal combustion engine, all provide models for our understanding of the body and the mind.

Most common of these contemporary myths are those of the *machine*-body, and the body as a system of pipes and tubes.

For many people, the modern body is seen as a hive of busy, industrial activity,, a productive machine of muscles and flesh. It is a walking, soft machine in an armature of bone, with mechanical organs and muscular gears. Its movements are coordinated by electrical impulses that flow from its computer brain, leaping like sparks from synapse to synapse, along the networks of nerves. It is powdered by nutritious fuels, and by high-octane beer or caffeine, pumped around the organs and limbs by that sabot-shaped engine throbbing within the chest.

Of course, this new body needs to have regular check-ups to ensure its roadworthiness. It needs to be serviced, repaired, oiled and overhauled. Old or worn-out parts must be removed, and replaced by spare parts lifted off the shelf, taken out of their wrappings, and implanted by surgeons within the body.

The inside of this body is often conceived in the image of domestic plumbing. Many people think it is made up of a series of hollow cavities – called 'chest', 'stomach' or 'bladder' – connected with one another, and with the orifices outside, by networks of piping or tubes. Diseases are seen as 'blockages' of one of these long soft tubes – an artery, a vein, a bronchus or a bowel. Such blocked tubes must be 'washed out' by laxatives, drugs or catheters, while the 'furred-up' arteries of the heart need to be regularly re-bored, or even 'bypassed', by the mechanics of medical science.

Thus, overhauled and plugged in, fuelled and ready, the body becomes a walking, talking, belching automaton, a clever copy of a human being, a mechanical toy governed by a computer-like brain.

The power of the computer as a model of ourselves, and of how we think, has been well described by Sherry Turkle in her book *The Second Self*. Among the new generation of the computer age, she points out, the distinctions are now blurred between computer and person. These days many of us ask those two uneasy questions: firstly, 'whether people have always thought like machines,' and secondly, 'will machines think like people?'

In his *Man the Machine*, the scientist Frank George answers both of these questions in the affirmative. 'Man is a machine,' he writes, 'who stores the information he collects and then utilizes that information in an intelligent way.' Such information, collected by the senses, is then stored inside the mind, that 'huge reference library' within the skull. Furthermore, man is the template for the computers we construct. This 'man-machine is made in man's image largely because man makes it, and he is copying – or trying to copy – himself.'

We are witnesses, writes George, to the birth of a new species, not a biological one this time, but a *'machine species'*. Advanced computers, vessels of 'artificial intelligence', have now appeared that could replicate, even improve upon much of what human beings can do. Somehow, faced with the arrival of these brilliant competitors, our own intelligence seems sparse, even strangely artificial.

Like Freudian theory, computer-talk has gradually entered popular discourse. In the age of computers and information technology, ideas, feelings, and the webs of memory have become merely the 'software' of the human spirit – a set of ghostly patterns within the soul. Now the brain is a structure of microchips, and the face and its features a Visual Display Unit, glowing with muscles and skin. People can now be 'programmed' or 'de-programmed', words can be 'processed', even memory becomes a matter of 'bytes', capacity or floppy disks. In this computer way of thinking, all of the past can be erased, stored, copied or edited – even though this abolishes along the way the sense of narrative, the pentimento of earlier experiences, and that rare sense of a personal moral history.

A man lies ill in a hospital bed, at the centre of a circle of solicitous machines. Without any effort, his sick body will give birth to a dozen descendants. With the machines as midwives, his suffering and pain will produce a new generation of patients that will outlive him, tiny things that flap and crackle in the air, as they are passed or crumpled from hand to hand, around the whitewashed ward.

These new offspring of the man are little squares or strips of paper, mute rectangles of plastic or celluloid. They are the graphs and photographs of his disease; the charts, tables, rows of significant numbers that measure his physiology; the printouts of his blood tests; the zig-zag tracings of his heart and lungs; and the mystical glances of the X-Ray machine.

The man watches as they are handed around and pointed or peered at, sighed over by the head-shaking doctors and nurses clustered about him. He feels lonely and abandoned as they lavish their tender attentions not on him, but on a thin strip of electro-cardiogram paper, a jagged-edged strip torn off a long roll, like a piece of toilet paper for a leprechaun.

As he lies in the bed, the sick man realizes with terror that all the colours and complexities of his life are being drained away. In the hospital he has been abstracted, translated by the medical machines into an arcane Cabala of numbers and graphs. He has been shrunk to the molecular level of his enzymes, to the size and number of his blood cells, the gasping capacity of his lungs, the electrical waves of his broken heart.

In the fluorescent, aquarium-like glow of the Intensive Care Unit, his body screams this knowledge every second of the day. The doctors listen intently, but they cannot hear him. They can only hear different sounds, whispered in a different language, somewhere inside his body – hidden, secret things that are happening in his blood-stream, or in the muscle fibres of his heart. Only his constant companions, the monitoring machines, are able to hear what he says. Gathered around his bed, they mumble among themselves in reply, beeping and buzzing in a worried dialect of dials and digital displays, like the underwater language of dolphins or whales.

Listening to their talk, he becomes a witness to his own metamorphosis. He has become an animated life-sized doll, with a tape-recorded cry implanted inside its head. Stripped of his clothes and ideas, his religion and kin, and all the other markers of his social self, he has become like that little writing automaton of Pierre and Henri-Louis Jacquet-Droz.

When the levers of Medicine are pulled, he becomes mute – his body only able to scratch meagre, disembodied messages onto the pieces of paper that they lay before him.

Later he begins to understand that a second, more subtle metamorphosis has also taken place. That his new mechanical body has become an oracle, for he has been turned from Man into Message, into an idol speaking in the clipped tongues of statistical science.

The doctors have plugged their powers into his body, and now – almost like sorcery – the body of the automaton talks back. They listen with veneration to the pronouncements of the idol they have created. Whispered into the ears of the metal high priests, the data flows swiftly onto the paper printouts, and its glow lights up the oscilloscope screen.

The sick man's conversion into an anthropomorphic machine, like our long fascination with mechanical dolls and automata, is the linear descendant of idol worship. Idolatry is not merely the worship of a tangible metaphor, the repository of a community's beliefs and values. By a circular route, it is also a man's worship of himself, or rather the narcissistic celebration of his own creativity. This is the secret allure of the idol, and of its many descendants. Constructed of wood, metal or stone, they are really a mirror, a projected image of our inner selves, and our ability to shape the natural world and its products into human form.

Turning an ill man into an automaton, regarding his body as a mechanical object, servicing his wounded heart like an exhausted engine, repairing his lungs like a fickle machine – are all strategies in the denial of death, the freezing of time. The Medusa machines that surround him monitor his internal mechanisms; but they also convert his life into fiction, into a curious form of abstract art, drawn in figures and graphs. Like medical documentary films, they turn human suffering and the biological fate of man into cultural artefacts, ritual creations of diagnostic science.

91

In our hospitals, we stare into the mirrors we have built, and listen closely to the electronic hum of their computerized oracles. Wired up in the ward, a human physiology carries on an electrical dialogue with a cardiac monitor machine, a complicated discourse of beeps, tracings and flickering lights. But somewhere in the background, among all the static, we think we can hear another sound – a thin silent one, like the invisible breathing of a hidden dwarf. It has that subtle resonance, almost a living vibration, that seems to surround all idols, automata and anthropomorphic machines. In some perverse way, they have their own independent life force. Sometimes they seem more human, more alive than the human beings who have created them.

For an idol is more than a solitary image. It is always a collective metaphor, an ideogram of all our thoughts, a mental phenomenon made suddenly visible. The worship of the diagnostic machine in the name of healing, and the mechanical model of the human body, both reveal the ironic paradoxes of modern society, and the folly at the heart of its medical science.

In this cul-de-sac of medical history, the door to the laughing room is always locked, or held against us. Inside it hide the three ciphers of the modern world – a silent man, a disembodied grin, and the vivid, abstract colours of a chuckling machine.

Outside the door, the woman has stopped sobbing. Birds gossip again in the trees. Overhead among the clouds the big-bellied Boeings fly, like huge whale-machines swimming through the sky.

Still the old man lies slumped on the floor, like a marionette forgotten between performances, mute testament to the artistry of its great creator.

And then slowly I realize that although he is not breathing, and his heart has stopped beating many hours ago, the man is not yet completely dead. Some echo of his life still remains.

I see the faint flicker of its colours passing across his face, the waxy skin reflecting the television screen, like a dream fading in the early morning light. Carefully I put down my medical bag, and slowly I walk over to the set to switch it off. There is a click as the colours fade to a small, glowing spot on the screen, a vortex into which the last laughs of the crowd spiral and disappear.

As I unplug the television, his life-support system for so many years, I feel uncomfortable, almost ashamed.

For some reason, difficult to define, disconnecting that machine feels like euthanasia, even like murder.

CHAPTER 7

✧

A Bridge of Organs

The woman leaning across the room towards me from the floral settee is tall and peroxided, and about forty-eight years old. They tell me that she is divorced, with two children, and a generous alimony.

Now she is relating to me, once again, her latest tale of woe. This time it is her stomach that is 'playing up', and she describes in intricate detail – clenching and unclenching both her fists – how after every meal it 'grips' and 'twists' and 'clutches' her from within. Last week it was a rash, invisible to everyone except herself. A few weeks earlier it was the turn of her heart, 'thumping' and 'banging away' at the walls of her chest like a small prisoner, desperate to escape.

Now she lives alone in this small suburban house, furnished as a sort of miniature Versailles, with a tiny pond built in its coiffured lawn, at the centre of a circle of stone statuettes. Seated in her lounge among pink silk cushions and velvet drapes, with gilt-framed reproductions on the wall, and serried rows of imitation antiques, she is describing to me the details of these latest symptoms. And all the while she is exchanging a thin cracked smile over my head with a collection of small porcelain shepherdesses clustered behind me at the very centre of the long marble mantelpiece.

As she speaks, I find my attention wandering easily away from her and her sing-song woes, past my black medical bag resting on the carpet, and across to the striped wallpaper and

94

the spindly-legged antiques. Everything in the room is of purple and gold, and all of it seems to be shimmering – though it is only half-way through the day – in the light of electric chandeliers hanging from the ceiling. Glittering under their many light bulbs, the whole scene seems borrowed from a distant nightmare of Marie-Antoinette.

I am fascinated by her nodding profile in the mirror hung on the wall. Slightly distorted, as if under layers of water, the reflection of her face in the glass is that of a Harlequin mask, a *commedia dell'arte* of colours and shade. Even at a distance, it is easy to make out the thick layers of her make-up, the falsity of her eyelashes, and the fibre-glass fingernails that scratch nervously under her chin. Everything about her is theatrical, everything in the room is like a set of painted props or paper scenery. Even her smile, one can see, is only an expensive creation of ceramic and gold. I watch those rows of dental guillotines as they rapidly rise and fall. These are the same ceramic blades with which she decapitates over forty cigarettes a day, spitting their lipsticked filter tips out of the car window, and into the passing wind.

Almost every day, she tells me, she is forced to run in sudden panic to the gold-edged bathroom, under attack once again from either her 'nervous stomach' or her 'irritable colon'. Driven to distraction by the malice of her digestive system, she searches frantically for her pills in the mirrored cupboard, rattling the rows of bottles on its little glass shelves. Like the books on a library shelf, each bottle can tell its own, particular tale. One tells of her insomnia, another of her migraines, and others of her nervous rash and her nervous tic. Every day, she says, terrified thoughts flee screaming from her head down into her stomach, and there metamorphose into waves of acid that burn and ulcerate her from within.

To those who have known her – family, friends and doctors – she seems to be like someone at the centre of a physiological civil war, in continuous conflict with her head, skin, bladder and bowels. She appears to feel assaulted, violated by different parts of her body, by the shape of her breasts and buttocks, even by the wrinkles that have crept all over her face. Over the years her friends have watched with a certain sad fascination the extensive re-modelling of her breasts and face. They have seen how four of her organs – her womb, her gall-bladder, her appendix and her tonsils, as well as numerous warts, bumps and blemishes – have all fallen victim to the surgeon's knife. Faced with her many aches and pains, she has been tested and probed, scanned and scoped, biopsied and X-rayed by hospitals throughout the city. She has been cut open several times, and then sewn together again – but each time the baffled surgeons have declared her organs unexpectedly innocent.

Almost everything about her house and its decor, and the blush on her cheeks is reproduction and false. And everything about her symptoms is bogus too, I am thinking, as I walk back towards the car carrying my bag.

In the taxonomy of medicine such a woman would usually be called a hypochondriac, or a malingerer, or a manipulative neurotic. Some doctors might even label her a sufferer from that unusual psychiatric condition, the 'Munchausen Syndrome', and say that she has become one of those sad, mad people – each one a tireless practitioner of partial suicide – who drift from hospital to hospital, their bodies adorned with fake symptoms, in the eternal search for a surgical cure.

But perhaps, in a symbolic sense, she is something more. For there is something oddly moving, almost Biblical about her, and the way that – in order to appease the dark gods of her psyche – she has sacrificed one organ after another on the altars of medical science. By now the surface of her body is criss-crossed with a complex filigree of these surgical scars, like a secret message written in cuneiform, or the parchment map of an ancient country. Among this soft cartography of flesh one can still make out the faint traces of wadis and caravan tracks, and the untidy rows of cicatrized hills, cut here and there into the white skin of her abdomen. For many years this body of hers has been the theatre of an unusual but archaic cycle of sacrifice, and an altar of her obscure immolations.

Back at the medical centre, flipping through the pages of her thick medical file as it rests heavily on the desk, I see that this woman is notorious in the area, the bane of all her previous doctors. On page after page their scribbled comments sneer at her, describing her as a 'heart-sink', 'resistant' or 'fat-file' patient, and pray that soon she will go elsewhere.

Her tale, recounted in the cool clinical language of her medical notes, tells how for almost a decade she has lived as if devils indigenous to her psyche, and some originating from her outer life, have come to possess one organ of her body after another. By some curious alchemy she has seemed to absorb all the traumas of her personal life into herself, to *embody* them into the cells and enzymes of her own body. Each part of her body in turn has become the container of all her unhappiness, a locked box of her suffering and pain.

Slowly over many years she has assembled these pieces of her pain together, and from them built a bridge to the outer world, a bridge constructed entirely of wounded organs. And now and again she has sent her screams of flesh and pain running across it, and waited anxiously for a reply, for any sign of the returning tip-toe of love. But each time nothing has happened. No one has ever returned, and her screams have died unanswered in the air. That bridge, it seems, leads nowhere in particular, except into the rooms of certain expensive doctors — suave medical mercenaries from Harley Street, each one a self-proclaimed specialist in some arcane malady. With their platoon of faithful assistants, they have been pleased to act as the centurions surrounding her on her personal Golgotha. In the deepest myth of her mind, some parts of her – whether they are innocent or guilty – must regularly die, crucified on a surgical slab so that the rest may live on, free of sin.

You can trace this bridge of her sacrifices all the way back and up to the Mount of Moriah, that more ancient ancestor of the hill of Golgotha. She has read – in Chapter XII of the Book of Genesis – how, at the command of his God, Abraham was willing to sacrifice his beloved son Isaac as a burnt offering. And she has read further, as, with hardly a pause, Abraham 'stretched forth his hand, and took the knife to slay his son'. And she has wondered at how, in the very last second of that famous tale, with Isaac bound on a hot wooden altar and the late afternoon sun reflected on the knifeblade, a sudden silence fell on the mountainside. All one could hear then was the whimpering of the bound child, and the swallowed sob of his father, and the cries of a buzzard wheeling high in the desert air. Then all at once, there was the *deus ex machina*. Satisfied by this demonstration of faith, Abraham's God sent him a ram, the one 'caught in a thicket by his horns', as a locum sacrifice. Isaac's life was saved – but was it really? What of the boy's future? she still sometimes wonders, what of the man he grew up into? – someone who would always carry the irregular scar from his father's shaking hand, cut deep into the carotid arteries of his psyche. Could he ever recover, he who was once saved only by an invisible voice, and the random arrival of a ram? Did he perhaps not suffer forever from some sort of 'Post-Traumatic Stress Disorder', with nightmares and flashbacks year after year, and a permanent phobia of knives, hot hillsides, father figures, and a certain species of ram?

Millennia later, here in this suburban desert, she has become both boy and ram, and she is also the knife, and the hillside, and the hot sun, and the father Abraham living with the memory of what he almost did, and why.

In the apparent autonomy of her organs, and in their malevolence towards her, the patient I call the Lady of the Bodily

Sacrifices represents something quite new: a novel and para-doxical type of body. This new body, emerging all around us, is a reflection of the individualistic societies in which we live. Increasingly we have come to view it in the same terms as the nation state in which it lives – as a sort of small 'society', sealed off from its neighbours by a border of skin. It is a composite of sentient and independent bodily parts, each with its own needs, dislikes, behaviour and personality. Some of these parts can even be hostile to one another, or to the person who carries them around. Temporarily assembled within its mobile borders, this new modern body consists of a crowd of unconnected strangers, living and squabbling in a community of flesh.

Within the body, each of these many 'citizens' has its own functions, its own rights and obligations. When necessary, each can vote its displeasure by causing specific symptoms or pain. In such a somatic democracy, the *health* of a person comes to be seen as a balance of interests, as an equilibrium between the needs of the various organs, cells, and fluids – just as it is in the wider body politic.

Implicit in this view is the conceptualization of disease as a form of unlawful 'dissent'. Thus modern diagnosis becomes the search for a dissident or anti-social organ, and its ritual accusation by medical technology. Ironically, as human ex-ecutions and euthanasia decline in the Western world, so its surgery makes possible the scapegoating, and execution, of the wounded or unwanted parts of our own bodies.

The border of the self is no longer the skin, the shape of the body no longer just the outline in the mirror, and the story of an individual body no longer just an autobiography.

'Spare-part' surgery has helped to breach the boundaries of the solitary self. The bits and parts of 'you' that are now 'non-you' – the ones that were borrowed from other people – will link you permanently to them in a new kind of way. Surgically inserted within the body, they will undermine the sense of a traditional, self-contained *communitas* of organs, confined within its own boundaries. They will dislocate the individual's sense of personal space, and of somatic time.

For each transplanted organ carries its own, unique life-history, and its own genetic autobiography – one that stretches all the way from its cellular birth and embryonic adolescence up to the full flowering of its adult organ-hood. In transplant surgery, one life-history is sutured into another, and within the body of the recipient the tributaries of a different time, and a different place, now flow together.

As he leaves the hospital after the operation, his face bloated with steroids, the transplant patient will carry forever – somewhere within his own skin – these hidden narratives of another life and of another death.

In Western culture – that traditional site of the cult of Individualism – the organs of the human body have long been seen as individuals, as entities with their own 'personalities'. Many body organs, for example, have accumulated their own literature and legends, and even their own theology. In these writings they are often described as if they were living beings, floating free from the human bodies that they inhabit. Even after death, they are commemorated in the posthumous worship of human relics – like those sacred bones and hearts of Saints in European cathedrals, or the pickled brain of Dr Albert Einstein.

Most famous of all these individualized organs is the Heart. In the pages of literature and theological history, it has long had its own special chapter.

Theological hearts have been prominent in Europe from at least the twelfth century onwards, when a cult of devotion to the Sacred Heart of Jesus began to develop. Over the centuries it has grown steadily, and many hundreds of prayers, poems and canticles have been dedicated to it – 'Through the Heart's wound, I see its secret,' wrote an early devotee, St Bernard, Abbot of Clairvaux. One of the first and most

famous apparitions of the Sacred Heart was seen by St Lutgarde d'Aywiers, while St Catherine of Siena saw hers in
1370. St Teresa of Avila, canonized in 1622, saw in a vision
her own heart, pierced by a burning golden arrow, shot by
an angel. 'Let my heart be pierced, oh Jesus,' cried St Francis
of Assisi, 'by that blade which transfixed Thy heart.'

Over the centuries, the Franciscans, the Dominicans and
later the Jesuits have added to this devotion to the Sacred
Heart, and by the seventeenth century prayers to the hearts
of both Mary and Jesus had been combined. On the recom-
mendation of his 'Congregation of Rites' in 1765, Pope
Clement XIII advocated the institution of the Feast of the
Sacred Heart, and the universal character of this feast was
proclaimed by Pope Pius XI as recently as 1928. The cult of
the Sacred Heart is commemorated in Montmartre in Paris
by the beautiful Basilica of the Sacré-Coeur.

Literature is full of a more secular type of heart – like that
of the Earl of Gloucester in Shakespeare's *King Lear*, whose

> flaw'd heart –
> Alack, too weak the conflict to support! –
> 'Twixt two extremes of passion, joy and grief,
> Burst smilingly.

Other literary hearts are like small excitable barometers of
love, passion, courage and will. In novel after novel they are
prone to leap, sink, jump or fall at the very words or glance
of a lover. Some of these hearts are described almost as fragile
balloons, liable to become so inflated with emotions that –
with a wild bang of pain – they can suddenly burst apart. In
the pages of romantic fiction, heroes and heroines are often
'heart-broken', 'heart-sick' or 'heart-sore'. Their thoughts
and emotions are 'heart-felt' or 'heart-rending'. They suffer
sad hearts, sore hearts, sick hearts, leaden hearts, burst hearts,
hearts full of sorrow or of joy. As you breathlessly follow
their fate, on page after page, these many types of heart

101

come to seem like little spherical people, full of their own independent life and loves, some even capable of outliving their human hosts. In that Edgar Allen Poe gothic masterpiece *The Tell-Tale Heart*, first published in 1843, this is exactly what happens. Poe tells how the disembodied heart of a murdered man lives on after his death – still beating quietly under the floorboards, but audible only to its murderer. It was 'a low, dull, quick sound –' cries the guilty one, in a shuddering confession that still sends tingles down our spines – 'much such a sound as a watch makes when enveloped in cotton.'

As far back as the fourth century BC, Aristotle had believed that the heart was more than just the seat of the emotions; he thought that it, and not the brain, was the true site of a person's intelligence. The brain, he speculated, was there mainly to prevent the heart from over-heating, by cooling it down with regular secretions of phlegm.

Thinkers of more recent centuries seem to have taken a cooler, less passionate view of the functions of the heart – as well as those of the brain. Gradually and firmly they have locked what we now call 'personality' and 'mind' and 'consciousness', and all thoughts, ideas and creativity, within that hard mobile suitcase they call the skull. Here in this bony box, say both the psychologists and the neurologists, reside the mysteries of individuality, the intricacies of the sense of self, the invisible ciphers of personhood.

In the nineteenth century, the phrenologists – those pseudo-scientific predecessors of today's neurologists – saw the bony surface and contours of the skull itself as a key to the qualities and passions of the individual, and believed that they could easily discover the mental powers, faculties and character of a man by examining the shape of his head. These qualities, they claimed, were revealed in the convoluted shapes and grooves of the brain itself, which were echoed in the bumps and dents of the skull bones around it.

These days, most people believe that the brain, and not the heart, is the actual site of intelligence, and of the sense of self – as well as the cardinal sign of humanness. Significantly, it is only in this present century, in the cerebral cities of our abstract society, that true and irreversible death is spoken of as '*brain-death*'. Despite the pleadings of literature, we no longer see a wounded or broken heart as the final event of an individual's life. But as they lie in their hospital beds, deep in the limbo land of an irreversible coma, their brains hardly functioning at all – the patients who are heart-dead but not yet 'brain-dead' are spoken of as if they had undergone a metamorphosis from one species into another; as if they were now evidence of a mysterious mutation of a human being into a *vegetable* – into a soggy, silent thing planted in a hospital bed, waiting quietly for the gardener's hoe.

Far away from the brain and the heart, in the deep south of the body, hide those other individualized organs – the Genitals – much-photographed stars of that basest of all art-forms, pornography. Spread across the Technicolor pages of porn magazines, they seem to have their own volition, their own secret and pagan personalities. Lit by the glare of the photographic lights, they behave like small furtive beings, exchanging with one another their rhythmic gifts of the night – and under the cold eye of the camera, glueing the staring strangers together, membrane to membrane.

Near the genitals lies the Womb, an organ that weeps tears of red disappointment every month of the year. In the past few years a woman's ownership of her own womb – already weakened by centuries of law, church, and medical technology – has become further diluted by the rent-a-womb of surrogate motherhood. For the first time in human history this process takes fertility, pregnancy and birth away from an individual woman, and shares them instead among a whole diaspora of wombs. And which of these scattered women, one may then ask, is the true owner of its tiny, growing guest? Is such a foetus a shared progeny now, or merely the temporary tenant of another woman's womb?

Though the womb is the source of human life, and of its continuity, men have always felt ambivalent towards its powers. Some have feared the polluting power of its menstrual blood, while others – remembering that the Greek word for womb was *hystos* – have blamed it for causing hysteria in women, the so-called *furor uterinus*. Over the centuries, some men have even believed that the womb was not fixed in place, but could wander at will within the woman's body, causing illness or hysteria as it did so. In the seventeenth century, Doctor Jean Libault wrote a description of how the womb could be 'ascending, descending, convulsive, vagrant, prolapsed', and thus could constantly change its position. Perhaps blaming the *hystos* for hysteria is part of the reason why, in the age of feminism, epidemics of hysterectomies are sweeping through the Western world, and why so many wombs have recently fallen under the scalpels of male gynaecology.

The womb is not the only organ to be blamed for illness and pain: in different parts of the world, nations have blamed other organs for most of their maladies. The British, for example, have long blamed their bowels for many of their symptoms; some of them have feared the 'toxins' that would leak into their bloodstreams if they were constipated and not 'regular as clockwork'. The French, by contrast, have for centuries accused their livers of causing a variety of illnesses – and many still believe that over-eating and drinking could cause them to have a *crise de foie*.

Of all the organs of the body, the Skin is the largest, and in a way the most autonomous, as it lives its life largely beyond our conscious control. Depending on the stimulus, it can blush or blanche, sweat or tremble, be flushed with sex, or pale with fear. It is the blank screen on which we project all of our hidden physiological messages. And we can also mark it like a pale parchment, or shape it or clothe it, or inscribe on its surface our own complex signals of scars, tattoos, paint and jewellery.

The closest cousins of the skin, the main sense-organs – the Eyes, Ears, Mouth and Nose – also lead their own disembodied lives, but their role is that of the accredited representatives of mankind. They are there to communicate – not only with the outer world, but with the similar representatives of other bodies. To pass on messages between them by consular lips, by ambassadorial tongues, or by the sounds of a plenipotentiary palate. As they scan the environment for food, danger or love, these sense organs also link the human community in a complex spider's web of perceptions – woven out of the invisible strands of sound, touch, smell, colour, movement, posture and pain.

Disembodied organs live on symbolically in colloquial speech, and in the discourse of the modern body. In this 'organ language' of contemporary life, it is possible to be 'tender-hearted', to 'vent your spleen' (that repository of bitterness and spite in the ancient theories of Galen), to 'have a bellyful', to be unable to 'stomach something', to be 'hearty' or 'brainy' or 'yellow-livered'. All of these are bodily metaphors with an old lineage, symbolic of the ways we still relate to our own bodies, and then to one another.

For many people, organs that are diseased are often declared independent of the body that carries them around. In a study of 800 patients in New York, for example, Dr Eric Cassell has described how these patients *reified* their diseased organs – and the diseases themselves – into an alien presence. They spoke of them as if they were an 'It', something external and foreign to their healthy bodies. Thus they described how they were afflicted by entities they called '*the* tumour' or '*the* arthritis', while it was '*the* ovary' that was diseased – and never me, or '*my* ovary' or '*my* breast'.

Sufferers from psychosomatic conditions, more so than

105

other people, seem prone to think of their organs as somehow alien and uncontrollable, and not completely part of the 'self'. They describe stomach, chest, bowels or skin almost as if they were autonomous interfaces between their bodies and the outside world, as if these bits of their bodies had their own volition, or were partly controlled by other people, or by other events. 'The bronchial tubes close, tighten up on me,' says an anxious woman with asthma, 'so no air goes into the lungs. When I feel nervous, I can feel them tightening up.' 'A row can make me tighten up,' says another woman, also with asthma. 'You get anxiety, and that gives you an attack.' 'When I get uptight with my husband,' says a third, 'I feel a tightness in my chest and I know I'm going to have an attack.'

Unpleasant emotions – just like painful organs – are often spoken of as if they were separate, external entities, somehow 'invading' the borders of the self. We suffer from a 'panic *attack*', an 'attack of nerves', an 'attack of the Blues', or an engulfing 'wave of depression'. These evil emotions seem to enter us unseen, and silently take up residence within our bodies and minds. Those that are seen as 'antisocial' – like fear, rage, envy and hate – are the ones most often spoken of as if they were something separate, somehow not part of the idealized self-image now common in the Western world. This ideal, modern self is one which is forever youthful and fit – a happy, healthy, productive and autonomous self, a bourgeois paragon of self-care and self-control. There is no place in modern society for the ill, the unhappy or the ugly. For them, and for the sufferers from uncontrollable symptoms – such as sudden vomiting, diarrhoea, belching or pain – the responsibility for their condition must always lie elsewhere. Thus for the psychosomatic patient, owner of a fragile self-image, it is the stomach that is always 'nervous', the bowel that is 'irritable', the 'nerves' that are weak or 'shattered' – but never the individual himself.

'Anger, tension, hostility, fear, any kind of upset – I think of them as being crammed into my colon,' says a 30-year-old woman with an irritable bowel syndrome, in a study carried out in Massachusetts – as if these emotions and organs were not really part of her. She copes with her stomach pains by 'trying to monitor what's happening. By being in touch with what's inside before the colon knows. By using relaxations . . . Talking to the various organs. It helps.'

'I put negative feelings inside myself,' says another woman, with ulcerative colitis, 'rather than put them outside myself. Doctors often say anger gets stored in the colon . . . Once something gets inside of me it just bounces around inside of me until I can get rid of it. If I can catch anger while it's fresh and pound something, it'll out of me – or someone will help me get it out.'

Such unpleasant, disembodied and 'non-self' emotions and feelings – those 'invaders' of body and soul – are really the modern descendants of ancient devils, ghosts, dybbuks, and ancestral spirits – and of all the other invisible inhabitants of a parallel and mystical world.

In many traditional cultures, people 'possessed' by these spirits or ghosts have undergone a sort of alchemical transformation as their entire body – its organs, moods, posture and tone – was believed to make visible the intangible world lying alongside our own.

In Europe during the Middle Ages and later, there was a widespread belief in this parallel world, peopled with invisible imps and malevolent entities. In the European witch-trials of the sixteenth and seventeenth centuries, the imperceptible personalities of this hidden world were revealed to all who were present, as the gruff tones of the Devil himself issued from the mouths of terrified old women or pubescent girls, accused of the crime of witchcraft. Or they revealed themselves in the writhing, rolling bodies of people possessed by spirits in the medieval streets on St Vitus'

Day, their faces and limbs twisted into a complex arabesque of posture and snarl.

Even today invisible and powerful entities are believed to emerge in those religions or cults where people talk feverishly in the dialects of glossolalia, speaking to the world in unknown tongues – almost as if they were human radios, tuned in to some distant, extra-terrestrial channel. They also emerge in those unearthly accents of the spirit mediums, as they bend over their candle-lit table-cloths; or in the voices of shamans and healers, chanting in their trances of divination, in the Arctic, Africa or elsewhere.

Just as Western society sees itself as a collection of independent citizens, and the human body as a collection of autonomous organs – so do modern theories of the human psyche speak of it as if it were divided into several, independent parts. Many of the theorists of psychology, for example, seem to assert that unhappiness and mental illness result from an acrimonious debate between different parts of the self. Between, say, the 'Underdog' and 'Topdog' of Gestalt therapy, or the 'Parent', 'Adult' and 'Child' of Eric Berne's Transactional Analysis. Earlier this century, the psychoanalytic theories of Freud had described in detail the three parts of the human psyche, almost as if the three social classes of Viennese society were represented within the divided self – the primitive, proletarian Id, without any inhibitions; the practical, rather bourgeois Ego; and situated above them both, the high moral government of the Superego, stern arbiter of laws and of penalties.

In previous centuries, writers on the anatomy of the psyche had spoken more of the *soul* of the human being than of the mind. St Paul, for example, had described the three aspects of man as *pneuma* – or spirit, which was the divinely inspired life-principle; his *psyche* – or soul, the life of a man in which that spirit manifests itself; and his profane body or *soma* – the actual physical mechanism animated by the soul.

108

To the Jewish Cabalists of the fifteenth century, the soul itself had four unique, though interwoven levels: the *nefesh* – the everyday soul of the living body; the *ruach* – or spirit of that person, his 'experiencing soul'; the *neshama* – or rational soul; and the highest level of all, the *yechida* or One-ness – that part of the soul that merges indistinguishably into the Godhead.

But it is not only in industrial societies that the psyche is divided into several different parts. In Latin America, anthropologists have described how, even today, the people of Zinancantan in Mexico believe that the soul is divided into thirteen parts, each one flowing from the life-force of a previous individual. Thus they believe that all persons alive today are only composites of the spirits of unknown humans who have lived before. Not far away, in Panama, the Cuna Indians also believe that each person has many selves – no less than eight of them – each of which is linked to a different part of the body, while the supremacy of one particular part determines that individual's temperament. A romantic is one who is governed by the heart, they say, a thief governed by the hand, an intellectual by the head.

Unlike the disembodied, individualized organs of the Western world, or the divided selves of its psychologies, the traditional cosmologies of ancient Greece, China and India did not consider individuals, their organs or their emotions, as being independent of their owner, or of other people or the cosmos. But like the Western model, they too believed that the borders of the body were not just defined by its boundary of skin. In these ancient world-views, all the wider forces that control and comprise the Universe were also believed to be present within the individual body – and thus its organs and emotions shared in the same cosmic mystery as the sky, the trees, the mountains, or the stars.

In ancient Greece, for example, the universe was believed to be composed of four elements, Earth, Air, Fire and Water, each of which was associated with one of the four 'qualities', Hot, Cold, Dry and Moist. In the medical theories of Hippocrates, father of modern medicine, who lived in the fifth century BC on the island of Kos, and in the later elaborations of Galen of Pergamum, these four cosmic elements appeared within the human body as four fluids or 'humours', called by the names *sanguinis* (blood), *pituita* (phlegm), *chole* (yellow bile) and *melanchole* (black bile). Depending on their relative proportions within each body, these humours harboured the mystical power to determine that person's temperament and bodily form – thus making men either sanguine, phlegmatic, choleric or melancholic.

In the traditional religious system of Ayurveda in India, a similar continuity exists between the body and the cosmos. The five basic elements of the Ayurvedic universe were the *bhūtas*, called Ether, Earth, Wind, Water and Fire. When eating a meal, the food containing these elements was believed to enter the body, and there to be 'cooked' by the body's fires, before being converted into bodily refuse. Within the body, these elements were then refined even further to form the *dhātus* – the seven basic components of the body – which were flesh, fat, food juice, blood, bone marrow and semen. The five *bhūtas* are also the origin of the three *humours* of the human body, for inside the body the Wind element became flatulence, Fire appeared as bile, and Water as phlegm. In ancient India, and still today, Ayurvedic practitioners saw health as a harmonious balance, as an equilibrium of all these cosmic elements both within and surrounding the human body.

Over two millennia ago in China, in his *Classic of Internal Medicine*, the Yellow Emperor Huang Ti also described the basic syntax of the universe as a cosmic balance – but this time between only two contrasting forces. One, known as *yin*, was described as dark, moist, watery and female, while the other, called *yang*, was hot, dry, fiery and male. The organs of the body itself were divided according to these principles – and were seen as either predominately yin (such as the lungs, heart, spleen, kidneys and liver), or as yang (the intestines, bladder, stomach and gall bladder). The concept of 'health' was understood by the Chinese as a happy harmony between these two forces in the cosmos, as well as within the human body. As in Ayurveda, disease was seen as evidence of disharmony or a lack of balance. In this case, the excess of either force accumulated within an organ might have to be removed from it – in order to restore the balance – by using herbs or other remedies, or by the sharp needlings of an acupuncturist.

In the ritual killing of her organs, the Lady of the Sacrifices seems, in curious ways, to be trying to transcend the limits of the modern industrial body – that little productive island bounded by skin.

For, in a limited, secular way, she is trying to recreate a sense of equilibrium and cosmic harmony in both herself and her social milieu. Just as her organs have their own, often disruptive personalities, so she too has long been the most disruptive organ of her own family, and of her own community. Faced with their hostility and rejection, she has offered them the sacrifice of her organs – but not of herself. It is an act of partial suicide, but also one of propitiation. By offering bits of herself to others, she is using them as a gift of atonement, and as a bridge to others, and as a way of crossing over that bridge towards them. But the pathos of her life is that all bridges go in both directions. For by now much of the interior of her body is held hostage by her relationships with other people – friends, family, a daughter lost to California, a son to psychotherapy.

Painfully she lives her life among an overlap of selves, for, like those of many other bodies in this modern world, her organs have become the remote colony of another self – the outposts of someone else's empire.

★

The combat between the woman and her organs, and the civil wars between them, are symbolic also of an unusual and contemporary way of being. Her body is more than just a theatre of sacrifice. It is also a sponge to the events of the world beyond its personal frontiers. The conflicts of her organs are really an echo of the conflicts and cruelty around her – an *embodiment*, as it were, of all the chaos and discord spilling from newspaper pages, or seeping out of radios and television screens and into her life.

These conflicts of the modern world, brought to us daily by the media, are providing us with a new set of metaphors, and a new way of understanding – and experiencing – the inner feelings and functions of our bodies. Like the psycho-somatic lady, we too are learning to absorb, physically, the daily history of the modern world. Embodied within our collective skins – as our 'nervous stomachs' 'grip' and 'clutch' us from within – are some of the notable stories of the twenti-eth century: world wars and uprisings, social upheaval and civil unrest, hijackings and hunger-strikes, squabbling tribes of bones and tissue, riotous crowds of unruly organs.

One day, when she has finally run out of disposable organs, the woman in the false Versailles will suddenly fall, and shat-ter into a hundred different pieces, like one of the porcelain shepherdesses dropped from her high marble mantelpiece.

When that happens, someone else – either her family or friends or a doctor – will collect all of these pieces from the floor, and sweep them together, and then carry them away in a large black plastic bag.

And perhaps some other day, a few millennia later, an archaeologist browsing through the ruins of a pre-nuclear civilization will find some of these little porcelain pieces buried in a mound that he is excavating. As he puzzles over the jig-saw of fragments laid out across his desk – a delicate hand, a cracked smile, a tiny blushing cheek, two small feet standing in the centre of a corona of broken sheep – and tries to cross the mental bridge between now and then, he will wonder what these pieces really mean. Perhaps he will speculate whether they are all parts of the statue of a tiny, beautiful woman and her devoted flock – or whether they are the fragments of a votive image, broken in a lost temple long ago, in some obscure rite of sacrifice.

CHAPTER 8

✧

The Dissecting Room

One day – it is a warm spring day in the Cape – I visit the pathology museum of the Medical School, and take a stroll through the aquarium of horror. The room and what I find in it remind me of one of those febrile, Hadean landscapes of Hieronymus Bosch, with fires incandescent in the distance. The rows of exhibits, pickled in formalin, are arranged on dark long wooden shelves, each shelf forming an entire bottled bestiary. There are malformations and mutants of every type: headless, eyeless, mouthless, one-eyed, three-armed, single-legged. There are pairs of twins joined at the chest or the belly. There is a liver, a head, a brain, a line of garish tumours, a collection of breasts and testicles in suspended animation. Floating in cloudy fluid, in some of the bottles tiny wrinkled homunculi, born of the worst nightmares of Paracelsus, stare through me as I walk slowly past them. Most disturbing of all are the typed or handwritten labels stuck to each jar, or pinned to the shelf. Their captions are bland or ambiguous, as irrelevant as the news headlines of a natural disaster, or the subtitles on a foreign massacre.

It is a relief to break open the bottles, to tear off the labels, to engage the flesh at last with one's scalpel. Already I know the feel of the knife as it divides its way through dead tissue. In zoology I have already dissected my way up the evolutionary tree. I have cut up earthworms and cockroaches, lobsters, frogs, dogfish and long white rats. I have watched a starfish ovum and a starfish sperm mating, without any foreplay, on the cold square glass of a microscope slide. Now I am ready for people, for anatomy, for a year in the dissecting room.

It is a long tiled room, in a special wing of the building, with low fluorescent lights and big misted windows, through which we can see the slopes of Devil's Peak in the distance. The human remains lie on symmetrical rows of high stone slabs, while clusters of white-coated students sit on stools around them. Tutors move among the slabs, pointing, advising, cutting. There is the clink of scalpel on skull and bared bone. The greasy pages of someone's *Ellis's Anatomy* lie opened on a nose, a chest, a forehead. There is a shrill laugh somewhere in the formaldehyded air. On all sides you can hear the low Latin murmur, the catechisms of dissection – 'latissimus dorsi, flexor pollicis longus, serratus anterior, the inferior vena cava –'

There, in the dissecting room, lie the stories of our society. There are the fuller bodies of the white philanthropic donors, and the thin and ravaged remains of the vagrants, the derelicts and the coloured paupers. The bodies on the slabs are black, or brown or a greyish-pink. There is no *apartheid* among the dead in our dissecting room but, clustered at one end, the coloured students – barred from ever touching naked white flesh – are permitted only to dissect the bodies of their own kind. In yet another room nearby, most of the women students lean over stripped human forms, free of the embarrassment of our presence. We cut and slice, we compare our bodies with one another. Someone plays cricket with a disembodied arm and a rolled-up handkerchief, but no one keeps his score, and the game quickly dies. Another group find themselves dissecting their old mathematics teacher, and remembering their examination grades, they reduce his ovoid frame with their scalpels to a more satisfying and

115

simple geometry. Others explore the bodies of naked strangers, stroking nudity for the first time in that long icy room.

All our dismantling is a true echo of the South African world outside the medical school. In our dissection we are imposing with our scalpels a kind of *apartheid* on the body, a splitting of the whole into named parts. We are breaking down into artificial categories something that had once had a living and organic unity. And in dismantling the human image, we are also dismantling ourselves. As well as these cadavers, something else will have to die, a coherent sense of what is human, an ancient shape in the mind.

In a small lecture theatre, between our dissections, the anatomy assistants bring in on white enamel plates a series of already dissected bodily parts. Some are wrapped coyly in damp white cloths, others are bare on the plate. There are skulls and bones, a hand with open tendons, a leg, an ankle, a steak-like cross-section of the hip, the abdomen or the thigh.

Lying raw in front of us, with the acrid smell of their preservative drifting up through the tiers of students, there is something shocking, but also comical, about these surrealist objects. There is horror in their violation of the human form, but they are also ridiculous. A nose, lying alone on the plate like a triangular snail. An ear, juxtaposed with an ankle. A hand and a spleen, sharing a plate. A head split cleanly down the middle, a Divided Self with half a nose, half a mouth, one baleful eye staring up at us, a solitary ear, half a brain and only half a silent tongue. Am I the only person in the room at that moment with a sudden headache, a scimitar of pain in the centre of my forehead, and a volcano of giggles rising inside of me?

It is curious, at first, to see how these slices and shapes mimic the illustrations in our anatomy textbooks. There is the same cut, the same angle, the same bisected female torso, the abdomen sliced through at the same level of the waist, the heart cut open between the ventricles just as on page 121. There are the branchings of the carotid artery, the nerve webs of the brachial plexus, the horizontal slice through the moist grey brain, the pelvic bone with muscle attachments painted on it in a dark blue ink. Nature is trying to imitate art here, but it is difficult to make the connection. How can one relate damp grey flesh to the gaudy painting, half a head to the coloured cartoon of a medical illustrator?

The afternoon is late. We have seen too many slices. The shuffling and the note-passing rise wavelike over the lecturer's voice. Now there is the temporary relief of fiction. A plaster manikin is wheeled in, a painted model of organs or systems, of cranial nerves, arteries, or the contents of the chest. Or they bring in a full-size plastic skeleton, Made-In-Japan, or a chart of the eyeball or the inner ear to hang on the wall. Now book and chart, model and sketch nod agreement to one another, and for us there is some deep peace in this. For an unusual moment the world seems right again, some dissonance has gone, and around me the chorus of a hundred ballpoint pens scratches their Amen.

In the dissecting room we come to realize the true paradox of anatomy. For the real agenda of dissection is the taming of Death, or rather the fear of Death. Because of this, we are asked to perform impossible alchemies. We must turn the cadaver into a three-dimensional textbook, a limited edition of tissues and organs. To do this, we must transform a dead body into the creation of a living body. The cadaver must become raw clay or pigment, the medical student a special type of performance artist. Our task is to create, or rather re-create, the body as a public sculpture, or as a series of sculptures. We must give to the body a posthumous life, through the rebirth of its parts. They must be reborn as *objets d'art*, as named, labelled, living commodities.

But in turning a body into a soft book, we are doomed to

117

be copyists. We are fakers who can only reproduce in cut flesh the abstract aesthetic of the anatomy book, with its lonely limbs and organs. Our signatures must remain hidden away, somewhere inside ourselves. In taming death, we have also tamed the anomalies of life.

Later that year, in the basement of the dissecting room, I understand these linked processes of dissection and creation, and why art has long been twinned with anatomy. As far back as the fifteenth century, the great artists of the Renaissance – Leonardo da Vinci, Michelangelo, Raphael and Dürer – were also anatomists, serious students of the human form. Da Vinci is known to have dissected at least thirty human corpses himself, besides many animals and birds. In his notebooks there are drawings of hearts, muscles, bones, nerves, and of a uterus split open like a walnut, to show the tiny foetus crouched inside. It was later, in 1543, that the first great textbook of anatomy appeared, that prize of dissection art, the *De Humani Corporis Fabrica* of Andreas Vesalius. Among his 300 illustrations are the famous full-page woodcuts of 'muscle men' – men stripped of their skin down to an elaborate underwear of muscles and tendons. Like mannequins on a catwalk, they adopt affected poses in Arcadian landscapes, among a tableau of rocks or trees or classical ruins. Some hang from gallows, their limbs provocatively splayed to show the muscle insertions of the limbs and trunk.

Other woodcuts show complete adult skeletons arranged in anthropomorphic postures. One skeleton leans in a Hamlet pose over a marble tomb, his tibias and fibulas crossed, and holds a solitary skull in his bony fingers, with his facial bones arranged in a thoughtful look as he contemplates the skull's familiar rictus. These collages of bones seem alive, they seem to have thoughts and ideas, often they are uncertain or sad. As they pose and strut through the tableaux, the skeletons and the muscle-men seem unaware of the fact that they are dead. Vesalius, like a true anatomist, has forgotten to tell them. Thanks to him they have been blessed not only with no imagination, but also with the amnesia of the recently deceased.

Other posing skeletons and muscle-men appear in the anatomical texts of the seventeenth and eighteenth centuries, but only appear in full flesh colour since 1746. In a book by Robert Knox, *Great Artists and Great Anatomists*, published in 1852, the author criticized those who drew these dissected muscle-men as though they were alive. Instead of drawing such a 'galvanized corpse', they should follow the lead of da Vinci: 'Draw the dead as dead – the living as living; never depart from the truth.' There was to be no confusion, on the page, between the two inevitable states of humanity. But the ambiguity remains: as we sharpen our scalpels, and glance at the textbook, both galvanized corpses and lonely organs compete for our eye.

We still call such illustrated guides to the human body 'anatomical atlases', and that phrase is significant. Now, as much as in the sixteenth century, they are maps and warnings of foreign lands. And in another sense, they are maps of unknowable landscapes, of geographies we can never grasp, however accurate the cartography.

The book we study from, *Gray's Anatomy*, was first published in 1858, but by now much of it is modern art, abstract and surreal. The bones and the nerves and the organs are still there, but fewer muscle-men or skeletons strut across the pages. Now there are photographs and X-Rays and micrographs in bright colours. Within the big human body, there is that new tiny body, the Cell, alone or in its communities. Paintings of its inner anatomy, its organelles, mitochondria or nucleus, are scattered throughout the book. Drawn or photographed through the cyclopic eye of a microscope, they are complex filigrees of colour, dots, lines, spirals, bands, like the canvases of a Miró or a Klee. Between these paintings, solitary and disembodied organs drift among the pages, afloat on seas of text, drawn by their slow current into our minds.

Three years later, before a big examination, I feel the swell of that invisible current. The intern in a medical ward takes me aside, and points. 'There's an interesting spleen over there,' he says, 'third bed on the left.' I walk along the ward, among the rows of beds, and follow his finger. And there it is, just as he said, lying in the third bed on the left – an enormous, black, and gelatinous thing, five foot long or more, moist and oozing off the sides of the bed. Nothing but a huge black spleen lying on a hospital bed. But then you blink and rub your eyes, and look again, and the spleen has gone, buried beneath the striped pyjamas of a little worn grocer of a man, sleeping in the bed. A small, sighing man with a sore stomach, and an ominous zig-zag chart, like a range of high mountain peaks, pinned to the foot of his bed.

But now, early in our anatomy year, I still sit in the hot cafeteria between seminars, among the girls sweating in their thin summer frocks, and secretly stare into that drab, engraved diagram in *Gray's Anatomy* – the one entitled 'The Female External Genitalia'. Each time I read underneath it, with that same baffled joy, the description of the Vagina. 'The female organ of copulation', it says, is 'a fibromuscular tube lined with stratified epithelium.' A fibromuscular tube! It has a sound like Latin poetry, or a tantric rhyme, a moist mysterious opening of language and flesh.

In some of our other textbooks, too, there are curious and suggestive illustrations, especially of the upper parts of the body. They seem to show grey woodcuts of the necks and faces of quite ordinary men. But these are not the pictures of corpses. They are living faces, indolent, asleep, or staring out past you from within the page, even though neck or cheek is sliced open to show you the blue-painted veins, the yellow nerves, or the Disney-red arteries hidden beneath the skin.

There is something familiar about the expression on the

faces of these men. It is that same look of weary detachment that you see in the faces of the girls and the sailors in those smeared photographs, the ones with their limbs intertwined in a complex Cabala of flesh and tattoo. Something violent and invasive is being done to them, too, in the name of illustration. They too are being dissected down to their fluids and their hair follicles, their distended organs and pink mucous membranes.

Thus the dissecting room shows us the difference between erotic art and pornography, between human experience and the worship of parts. For the true parallel of dissection, as an esoteric form of performance art, is pornography. It is the same reduction of the human image into slices of helpless meat, ripped out of context. Whatever the caring aim of medicine, all this is only one stage beyond those vermilion cuts of meat you see hanging in a butcher's shop. It resembles rather the slices of meat on display in the big, fluorescent supermarkets. Here meat has become a daring, abstract form of art, in frames of white styrofoam covered with a cellophane sheet. Cows, sheep, pigs and lambs have all been reduced to priced and labelled exhibits, products of the avant-garde, in the long corridors of an art gallery. They are original oils by Francis Bacon, at a price almost anyone can afford. Like other forms of art, they are commodities to be bought, to be taken home, to be displayed to other people, to be cooked and then consumed.

One morning, I witness the actual birth of a muscle-man. The chief technician of the Anatomy Laboratory takes us down to the long icy room in the basement, with its jars and boxes, its obscure odours, and the several rows of steel trolleys.

On one of the trolleys lies the newly delivered body of an elderly coloured man. He is being prepared for the dissection room. I see he has some of the high-cheeked features of the indigenous peoples of the Cape. Somehow, a few resilient genes of the Bushmen and the Hottentots have survived the bullets and smallpox of the white settlers, right up to the present. He has not only the usual posthumous pallor, but also that shrunken look of poverty and malnutrition. He is a man who has eaten very little, for far too long, and now has a fallen face, and a thin, naked Belsen body. He lies alone on a metal trolley with bottles of a bright red liquid dripping down long plastic tubes, into his shrivelled tissues and his blood vessels. He reminds me of the comatose patient I had seen in the Intensive Care Unit of a hospital, but there are no nurses or humming machines around him, and from this particular coma he will not recover. While we are staring down at this old, ravenous body – this 'fresh cadaver' as they call him – the chief technician is stroking his curly white pubic beard and imparting to us, in a guttural whisper, some of the arcana of the embalmer's art. He tells us about the dyes, the fluids, the fridges, the special tissue preservatives, the little tricks of conservation that his colleagues can only envy. Then he sends us away, for coffee and chocolate milk in the cafeteria.

And when we return in the afternoon, we are witness to a marvel of perverse alchemy. In a few hours, the world has turned upside down. The Hottentot man is no longer dead, but now only asleep on the trolley, and very deeply so. With his tissues swollen with red embalming fluid, his emaciation has gone. The parallel valleys between his ribs have gone too, as have his sunken belly and thighs. His arms and legs are now the muscular limbs of a young, sleeping man. His cheeks too are plump, and of a good colour. Now he lies on the trolley, flushed and contented, like a man resting in the hot Cape sun on a park bench or a beach, after a full meal and a fine red wine.

He has become Art, a leather sculpture of a sleeping man. And in his fate I see another parable for South Africa. Behind the tanned skin of the farmer and the beach boy, a red embalming fluid has slowly replaced the human blood and the tissues. In the African sunlight it gives off a flush of permanence and health, but like the Hottentot it is the genesis of art, not of nature. It is only preparation for a lesson in dissection. A lesson that has just begun.

CHAPTER 9

✦

A Time of the Heart

Think of it as a small, round, flat machine made of a shining metal, a marvel of complex engineering.

As it travels swiftly through space, flying towards our ears, we can faintly hear through the intervening air the intimate whirr and click of its inner machinery. And when it comes nearer, and we can see it even more clearly, we begin to realize what a wondrous and enigmatic machine it really is, with its glimmering surfaces and smooth, impenetrable skin. Through the protective bubble of plastic or glass on one of its sides, we catch a glimpse of its luminous console of numbers and dials, a glowing display of its unearthly technology. Silver, steel, platinum and gold are the shiny textures of this curious craft, as with every beat of its metal heart it carries its solitary passenger inexorably into the future.

It is a craft built to travel through space, but also for a voyage through time.

In the streets of a certain modern city, a particular type of man or woman strides quickly among the crowds on the way to an appointment.

This person is middle-aged or less, and usually middle class: perhaps a manager in business or sales, the executive of a corporation, or a rising star in some big multi-national company. Or even, judging by the cut of the clothes, a politician, a professor, a lawyer or a doctor.

124

Let us consider an example of this type, as he sits anxiously in a waiting room, writhing and foot-tapping in his seat in counterpoint to the jerky tic of his hands and face, while glancing down repeatedly at the little time-craft strapped to his wrist. Suddenly, he realizes with horror that he is now late, very late, for his scheduled appointment, and that *time is being wasted*, precious time slipping away like quicksilver through his sweating fingers.

The circular image of his watch-face and its relentless hands fly swiftly into his eyeballs. A split-second later, and the worried impulses are speeding from his eyes along his optic nerves and into his brain. Somewhere in the antechamber of his mind, the alarm bells begin to ring. You are late! they ring, You are late! You are late! You are LATE! LATE! LATE!

Alerted by the din, the adrenal glands in his abdomen quickly secrete their two hormones – epinephrine (or adrenaline) and norepinephrine – into the bloodstream. Pumped around the body by the heart, these magical, alchemical fluids transform his organs instantly into an emergency posture of fight or flight.

In a state of high alertness, his eyes darting here and there, with their pupils dilated, he scans the room for danger or threat. Deep within his body, stores of high-energy glucose are released from his liver into the bloodstream – emergency fuel and food for his terrified physiology. His mouth has begun to dry up, his tongue sticks to his palate, his breath comes quickly in a syncopated rhythm, panting in pursuit of the racing beat of his delirious pulse.

Hastily on the surface of the body, the blood vessels of his skin contract, shunting their precious blood back into the body, and into its most vital organs – the heart, the brain and the kidneys. All over his now cold and clammy skin, hair follicles come rigidly to attention, and point their tiny javelins out at a hostile world. Meanwhile, way down south in the abdomen, all the sphincters are contracting, and the

125

serpentine movements of his bowels are frozen in terror, as they wait for the crisis to pass.

Faster, faster, and faster pumps his heart, faster and faster – You are late! You are late! Late!! Late!!! goes the beat – Pump! Pump! Pump! Pump! – pushing the pressure of his blood, the scream of his nerves, higher and even higher.

Suddenly, as the panic hormones shriek in a carousel round and around his brain, the door opens wide, and with a mumbled apology an older man appears, and ushers him quickly into the room.

During the interview, perched pale and sweating on the edge of his seat like a bulging bag of adrenalin, he struggles to squeeze his body and its business back into the shrunken container of the late appointment. He speaks quickly, urgently, clenching his teeth and his fists – as the words burst out of him in a gush of verbal lava, erupting from some tortured Mount Etna deep within his soul.

Some hours later, back at home, and after a brief bite and a nod to his wife and children, he is back at work again, poring over the forms, printouts and pocket calculators spread across his desk – joining or subtracting number to number, slicing or suturing them as the midnight hour rolls nearer. For now – as always – he has no time to relax, no time for his family or friends, no time even to sit and watch the television. For his life is spent in a regular oscillation between two brief aphorisms – 'Time is money,' he says one moment, rubbing his eyes and bending forward over the desk, and then adds with a yawn – 'and money is time.'

The cardiologists of contemporary medicine have called this curious, though common way of living a modern life the *Type A behaviour pattern*.

They describe the 'Type A' person as that familiar figure of modern life – quick, ambitious and competitive, always hyped-up and hostile, and obsessed with time and its many deadlines. Every moment of the day, these men and women feel the fraught sense of a shortage of time. Their lives are spent in an unending battle with the invisible constraints of the clock, and in a struggle to achieve more and more, in less and less time. Greedily they make use of every minute, every allocated second, before their account in that big bank of time runs out, and that great Bank Manager in the sky refuses to give them an overdraft.

We recognize them easily as the familiar 'work addicts' or 'workaholics' of the modern world, people who would suffer withdrawal symptoms without their daily fix of adrenalin or angst – who jog relentlessly along the pathway towards greater wealth, and yet poorer health.

Studies have shown that they are over twice as likely to suffer a heart attack, or some other dangerous heart disease, than other people – especially as opposed to their hypothetical opposite number, the so-called 'Type B'. This pleasant and placid individual, as described in the medical textbooks, is a relaxed and laid-back person, friendly and non-competitive, someone well satisfied with his status, and with a life centred mainly on the circle of his family and friends. Such people are often spoken of, in the medical literature, as if they were a sort of smiling, urban beach bum, indifferent to the constraints of clock-time, and to the siren calls of profit and social ambition.

The 'Type A/Type B' model of human behaviour, although it originates within modern medicine, can really be seen as a sort of moral parable of good behaviour versus bad. Yet like other parables from all over the world, hidden in its aspects of light and shade are always the seeds of ambiguity. For the society of today *rewards* the Type As and their cruel and self-destructive lifestyle. This frantic ilk become the leaders, the managers, the top executives, and the well-paid politicians and professors of the Western industrial world.

★

The Watch and the Clock are the two central ikons of this industrial civilization, and all of the modern world is their *iconostasis*. Nearly every adult carries such a little holy image strapped to his wrist, or hangs it – framed in silver or in gold – upon his wall. For generations the ikon has tick-tocked all around us, at home and at work, on the desk, the sideboard, the mantelpiece, and the dashboard. And gradually its familiar 'face' and 'hands' have given way to the luminous wink of a digital clock, flashing its oracular message to us in a cryptic, numerical language.

Every morning in the early blue of dawn, multitudes of its devotees rise yawning from their sleep, bowing before the sacred moon-face or the changing numbers of their ikon on the bedside table. Then, pulling on their clothes, and clutching their holy diaries, they rush wildly out to prayer, streaming out of their homes and houses in a synchronized surge of millions of bodies.

In this way, we are a culture of wrist-glancers and time-worriers. Almost every adult body now dances its daily *pas de deux* with the clock, and plays a physiological duet with the little machine tied to its wrist.

Of all the human bodies on planet Earth, it is those of us living in the Western half that have the closest relationship of all with this machine – as the regular beat of the clock forces its way into our cells and hormones, shaping the tempo of our heartbeat and breath.

In modern society, clock-time is the invisible matrix of everyday life. We live among its rhythmic beat as it infiltrates the mind with *zeitgebers*, those subliminal time-cues from the environment: the early-morning tringing of alarm clocks, the clatter of breakfast plates, the arguments of waking children, and the hoot-hoot of cars in the streets outside. And later in the day, there is the click and buzz of the factory clock, the news broadcasts on the hour, and every hour, and the late-afternoon cadence of elevators, doors slamming and cars revving, as the 'rush hour' of traffic begins to head back towards the sunset suburbs.

We live our lives submerged in the invisible fluids of time. Every day and every night we swim our way through it like fish, goggling at the world through its movable, liquid lens. We eat it and drink it, and drown in it eventually. But always we are unaware of it, until that unexpected final moment, when – for an instant, or perhaps for ever – we find ourself lying on a timeless beach, stranded and alone.

It was the anthropologist Edward T. Hall who first described the two types of time common in the United States, and in other parts of the Western world. Most powerful of all is what he termed *Monochronic* time – the public time of business and bureaucracy, of schedules and appointments. It is the time of men and management, of the sports and professions – a linear, sequential time of clocks, diaries and time-pieces. For those of us who live in monochronic time, time itself is seen as a ribbon, or a road, or a line that stretches inexorably from the past into the future. It is divided into little equal slices that we call 'years', 'months', 'days' or 'hours'. For us, every event and every moment has both a beginning and an end; and between the two one can do only 'one thing at a time'. These linear strands are woven into the fabric of our existence, moulding our perceptions and feelings, and our relationships with other people. All of our social life is dominated by appointments, by diaries and schedules, which slice up the seamless flow of life into little compartments, sealing off within them one person or more from the world outside. For Western people, wrote Hall, 'time is an empty container waiting to be filled.' The container moves along as though on a conveyor belt, and if time is wasted, the container slips by only partially filled, and the fact that it is not full is noted. Monochronic people assume that he or she is the only one who can fill those containers – with talk, work, play or other experience. They place a high, mystical value on speed, efficiency and deadlines, trying to achieve more and more in less and less clock-time, to fill to overflowing the time containers as they whizz swiftly by.

In industrial countries, monochronic or clock-time is above all a form of *order*, a type of discipline imposed from outside on the chaos of human life. We learn the beat and order of this time in infancy, with the schedules of feeding, and later from the bells and timetables of our schooldays. In the West, 'time is organization,' said Hall, for it is the invisible skeleton of industrial society – a concept very different from the Zen Buddhist philosophy of the East, where 'time springs from the self and is not imposed.'

The origin of this linear model of time, wrote Joseph Needham, lies in the cosmology of the Judaeo-Christian world, with its 'continuous linear redemptive process'. Such linear time was intrinsic to Christianity, with its belief in the progression from the *creatio ex nihilo* up to the Second Coming. For both Christianity and Judaism the entire world process could be seen as 'a divine drama enacted on a single stage, with no repeat performances'.

This spatial metaphor of progress or movement was woven into the writings of the philosophers of eighteenth-century Europe, whose belief in the perfectibility of man through his own efforts, and of a human Progress advancing through history, still influences our modern way of thinking. In the nineteenth century such ideas set the stage for theories of the linear evolution of the human species, and of civilizations, and they still influence many of our contemporary assumptions about 'developed' and 'developing' nations.

But even here in Europe and North America, millions of people – mainly women, the young, the elderly and the unemployed – still live their lives largely outside the cold control of clock-time. They live in another type of time – called *Polychronic* time – the more human, qualitative time, the time of people, and not of punctuality – and the time of doing things for them, and with them. Here tasks are completed only 'when the time is right', and not before. So food must be prepared for the palate or for friends, and not just for the clock – and social talk and human warmth are more important than diaries and appointments.

Time, to polychronic people, is not powerful or tangible enough to be 'lost', 'wasted' or 'spent'. It is neither a ribbon nor a road, but rather a *point* at which events or meanings or relationships converge. Polychronic people, wrote Hall, 'are oriented towards people, human relationships, and the family, which is the core of their existence'. They are involved in multiple tasks, and ties to other people; time and their life are in flux, and nothing is so fixed or cold as the inscrutable face of the clock. Thus polychronic time is the more private time of the home, not the public time of the world of managers or market places. Many women who work in the home live much of their lives in polychronic time, and so do many millions in rural areas of the Third World and elsewhere.

Hidden in the interstices between these two types of Western time – monochronic and polychronic – are other, unique times, each with their own special characteristics. Included among them are the heightened times of sex, prayer, illness or ecstasy; and the special zones of time occupied by those in certain occupations, such as farmers embedded in the cycles of the seasons, monks in the rituals of prayer, artists in the moments of sudden inspiration.

Millennia ago, the only dividers of time were the human life-cycle, and the cycle of the seasons – the ebb and flow of heat, fall, rain and snow. The only interruptions in these currents of time were the cyclical festivals of the pagan year – the festivals of harvest, spring, mid-summer and autumn. Then there were the early-winter festivals of lights, glowing in the dark of the long cold nights – early ancestors of those other candle-lit festivals we now call Christmas, Chanukah, and Diwali.

In the early Middle Ages, time in Europe became linked to the holy cycle of religious festivals. Saints' days, Lent, Christmas and Easter were the high peaks of the Christian year, often superimposed on the older pagan cycles of the seasons. At first the only markers of time were the church bells, their peals echoing over the fields and forests, as they signalled the times of devotion and prayer. From about the thirteenth century onwards mechanical clocks in public monuments and churches began to appear, also linked to the cycles of prayer. Later, in burgeoning towns all over the continent, other clocks were erected on town halls or towers, regulating the daily work-cycles of all their adult citizens. In the fourteenth century or thereabouts, personal clocks appeared – though at first they were only the bejewelled toys of royalty or the rich. By the mid-sixteenth century, there were clockmaker guilds in cities and towns all over the continent, making their mechanical clocks for the newly rich citizenry. In the seventeenth and eighteenth centuries, the notion was born of a 'universal clock', one that meted out the same single time all over the world, a time that was everywhere and the same. Thus Isaac Newton spoke of an 'Absolute, True and Mathematic Time' that was universal and invariable. This Newtonian thought, twinned with that of Descartes, created the idea of an ordered, mechanical, clockwork world – and in this image lie the metallic seeds of the Industrial Revolution.

For without clocks, there can be no industry, no factories, no organization of millions of workers. Thus the rise of the Western industrial world runs in close parallel with the apotheosis of the clock. In Britain, by the 1850s, those little time-craft, strapped to a wrist or dangling from a waistcoat chain, began to be seen in all parts of the country. For the first time, watches were mass-produced, and the beat of their tinny little hearts soon spread out into the population. Soon millions of bodies were synchronized, and linked permanently to those two Great Clocks of nineteenth-century industrial society – the schedules of the day and the work-week, and the timetables of the new-fangled railways spreading across the countryside.

With clocks beating their way into millions of bodies and minds, large masses of workers could be coordinated, and could be made to move here and there across the city or the factory floor, or drive tooting and hooting on schedule in the 'rush hours' of millions of buses or cars.

Within the factories themselves, the clock on the wall, or the siren on the roof, became a sort of mechanical foreman, tightly controlling the workers with its dehumanized beat, as it regulated the daily pace of their productive lives.

Running parallel with this rise of clock-time, there has always been the mystical emphasis on *numbers*, on the numerical worship of quantity, and not of quality – a way of thinking essential for industry, banking, book-keeping, and for the calculation of profit and interest.

The Type A individual, with his unique time-mania, is a sub-species of this modern Numerical Man – that worshipper of numbers and statistics, and devotee of the god of percentages. For his world-view too, clusters around that series of modern symbols we call 'numbers'. To such a man, these numbers are much more important than people, quantity always wins over quality – and the magic symbolism of a 'hundred percent' marks the only boundaries of his knowable world.

In the Western way of thinking, time has long been a tangible thing. It is odourless, colourless, tasteless and invisible, and yet we can almost touch it or feel it as it moves through our lives, or watch as it slips like hour-glass sand through our clutching fingers. In our culture, time is a complex symbol, a mnemonic of many meanings, whether we conceive of it as a ribbon or a road, or as a broad river rushing swiftly out of sight over the horizon, or as the consumer of man and all his fragile works. *Tempus fugit*, we say, and mourn its rapid flight, in fiction and in verse.

Swallowing down another antacid, as he glances down at his watch, the businessman knows that, as well as an invisible road, time is also an invisible *currency*, an unseen commodity, a thing to buy other things with. He knows that time can buy money, and money can buy time. And that profit can be turned into time, and time turned into profit, and profit into even more profit if invested rightly. In the daily discourse of his life, time can be 'spent' or 'invested', 'wasted', 'used', 'bought', 'taken', 'saved' or 'given'. It can be 'free-time' or 'spare-time', 'extra-time' or 'over-time'.

And in the corporation for which he works, time, wages, labour and productivity are all closely interwoven. More bonuses for him, and more profit for the firm – he knows – comes only from more goods produced, more goods ordered, more contracts signed, and all of this in a shorter and shorter time.

Most of modern American time, wrote J. T. Fraser, is just such an invisible commodity, but only when it is *present* time: for in American culture 'the past is useless, the future of interest only as a potentially better present.'

The sociologist Max Weber, writing at the beginning of this century, saw the theological roots of capitalism, and its profit perception of time, in the fertile soil of ascetic Protestantism, and in the Puritan ethic of the early United States.

Puritan writers of the seventeenth century, such as Richard Baxter, had preached the virtue of hard work, of continuous bodily or mental labour, but they had inveighed against 'the spontaneous enjoyment of life and all it had to offer'. Each man's work, or his 'calling', was his personal pathway to God and salvation – but only if this labour produced wealth or goods for the benefit of others. 'Private profitableness' was agreeable, but only if made with the purest of motives.

134

'You may labour to be rich for God,' wrote Baxter, 'but not for the flesh and sin.' Wealth was thus a danger for it might bring idleness and leisure, temptations of the flesh, and all the other distractions from the religious life. To the stern-faced Puritan, noted Weber, 'waste of time is thus the first and in principle the deadliest of sins. The span of human life is infinitely short and precious to make sure of one's own election. Loss of time through sociability, idle talk, luxury, even more sleep than is necessary . . . is worthy of absolute moral condemnation.' So time was valuable beyond measure, for 'every hour lost is lost to labour for the glory of God.'

By a century or so later though, something odd had happened to these images of American time, and their relationship to the pursuit of wealth. Both had undergone spectacular transformations. For now time had become a currency, a secular commodity stripped of most of its ethical and religious wrappings. In a canny essay published in 1736, called *Necessary Hints to Those That Would Be Rich*, Benjamin Franklin warned his readers that: 'he that idly loses five shillings worth of time, loses five shillings, and might as prudently throw five shillings into the sea.' And furthermore, he added, 'he that loses five shillings, not only loses that sum, but all the advantages that might be made by turning it in dealing, which by the time that a young man becomes old, will amount to a considerable amount of money.'

The medical model of the Type A behaviour fuses three of the central symbols of modern Western culture: *Time, Money* and *the Heart*.

Deep within the chest of the Type A man lies hidden the third of these three symbols of contemporary society – the metronome of clenched muscle, that little muscular machine that beats the inner rhythms of body and mind.

The two cardiologists, Dr Friedman and Dr Rosenman, who first described the Type A behaviour pattern, saw it as originating within 'modernity', and in those values of

Western culture that reward such materialist behaviour. To them, the stresses of modern life 'are of a variety never previously witnessed in any previous age of society'. Coronary heart disease, wrote Rosenman in 1978, is the 'twentieth-century epidemic', resulting from 'psychosocial factors that are unique to this century'.

But whether this is true or not, embedded in this model there seems to be a nostalgia for a pre-industrial Garden of Eden, for a 'Type B' world of patience and leisure, a slow and friendly childhood lived once in some far Arcadia of the mind.

This fear of modernity, and of its effect on the heart, is not in itself new. Back in 1897, the famous physician Sir William Osler had warned his colleagues that 'arterial degeneration' resulted from the 'worry and strain of modern life', and from 'the high pressure at which men live, and the habit of working the machine to its maximum capacity'.

These days, in that most modern of all nations, the United States, heart disease and the terrifying 'heart attacks' that it causes, still have their own symbolic significance, and have even acquired their own mythology – especially among middle-aged men. 'We even feel that we know who is going to get one,' writes Dr Eric Cassell, a physician in New York. '"If he keeps on going like that", we say, "he's going to have a heart attack." In our modern minds, heart attacks have a relationship to what we do, as if we bring them upon ourselves.'

Not all doctors agree with the Type A model of heart disease, and with its linear connections of cause and effect. For no one yet understands how one type of behaviour can break a particular heart, while another continues to beat free.

But in a symbolic sense, the model can mainly be seen as a type of parable, or as a metaphor of the many contradictions within the modern psyche.

The Type A individual – that driven, competitive man

who has made a Faustian pact with the ikons of Time – lives his life in a bizarre union between the ticker on his wrist, and the ticker in his chest. He is a walking paradox, a living symbol of social conflict – someone who is both social rebel and social conformist at the same time, and within the cellular structures of the very same body. On the one hand, he is a workaholic foot-soldier of the economic system, conforming to what Weber described as the ethos of capitalism – its 'philosophy of avarice' and 'the duty of the individual towards the increase of his capital, which is assumed as an end in itself'. But on the other hand, he is someone whose behaviour is *anti*-social, hostile and destructive to many of those he lives and works with, especially his family, friends, colleagues and employees.

He also stands at the intersection between many of the other conflicts of our modern life: conflicts between the values of the home, and those of the work-world; between the ideals of Benjamin Franklin, and those of the Puritans; between time as a holy service, and time as a currency; between time as a ribbon, and time as a point in human affairs; between quantitative and qualitative time; and between what the Greeks called *chronos*, or linear time, and *kairos* – the human, living time of seasons, goals, feelings and emotions. And somehow all of these many conflicts and paradoxes are embodied within him, carried about within his person, and within the microscopic fibres of his own particular heart.

He is the living metaphor of our times, one of those tragic heroes of Western society – the moral marionette with too many puppeteers – and thus a man whose fate is known and pre-ordained, by all except himself.

For the sake of all those around him, the paradoxes of his many lives must one day be resolved. And on that awaited day, when patient Fate cuts through his heart-strings, the hurrying marionette in the business suit will fall and fall and fall . . .

And many of the contradictions of our society will converge upon the fragments of a certain broken heart – beating irregularly like a damaged clock, in the depths of a certain chest.

One day between appointments, as he leaps from page to page of his crowded Filofax, he experiences – somewhere within his chest – a curious sense of dissonance. It is the pain of a deep disagreement, between the metal heart strapped to his wrist, and the clock ticking within his chest. Trapped by this painful and irregular argument, he gives a strangled moan, and clutching at himself, slumps slowly to the floor. For an elongated moment as he falls, he wonders whether finally this is the mugging that he has always feared – the 'attack' upon him by his own heart.

Some days later, lying in a hospital bed tethered to the machines and monitors of the Intensive Care Unit, at the hub of a halo of worried white coats, the heartsore man listens to the fragile beep-beep-beep of his heart echoing in the machines, like the call of an anxious bird.

Gradually he begins to realize that his suffering has been turned into parable, and that the hospital has become a sort of classroom for his moral improvement. As he listens to the murmuring of the doctors and nurses around him, he can feel himself falling down a vortex of social despair. To his chagrin he comes to see his heart attack as the inevitable result of his values and life-style – the bitter fruit of all the expensive trees he has ever planted. He learns that his pain is a punishment, for he has broken some of the subliminal rules of family and society, rules he has never known, or has long forgotten. But what rules are these? he asks himself again and again, tossing and turning in the hospital bed – with that deep, existential terror of the arch-conformist. He peers around him for an answer, at the rows of silent, broken men lying beside him – but no one will meet his eye, and no one replies, and in the room nothing can be heard except the worried buzz of the watching machines.

Some weeks later, the man emerges from the hospital into the arms of his family, chastened, fragile and pale. We told you it would happen, they seem to say silently; we told you it would all catch up with you. Be less competitive and less ambitious, and don't be so angry, warn the doctors. Forget about the clock, spend more time relaxing with your family, counsel the nurses. Try to learn to relax, forget about dead-lines – says the little booklet, handed to him as he leaves the hospital – stop competing, start delegating your responsibilities.

They drive him home in a sympathetic silence and, seated in the car around him, the family re-establishes for a while its sense of a shared and continuous life, free of the pull of factory or firm.

Sadly the man watches the rhythm of the advertising billboards, as they flash like Technicolor time-craft past the car window – Spend! Borrow! Spend! Borrow! – shriek the alternating signs – Earn! Invest! Spend! Borrow!

Slowly the sun sinks under the horizon, and an orange flame covers the sky, like the flames of a burning Filofax. Thoughtfully he sinks back into his seat, and with an ambiguous sigh twiddles the dials of the car-radio until a swirl of music fills the air.

Mile after mile, and the billboards are fading away, and in the darkening distance he catches a glimpse of the first stars being born on the horizon, just as they have been every dusk, ever since the world began.

For a brief moment, held gently between the fingers of day and those of night, he has a sudden sense that his life could still be different. Perhaps, as he watches those stars ascending, he can feel the timeless cycles of the ancient myths, and how they are still resonating within the fibres of his own body, and in the regular beat of its pulse.

NOTES

✧

CHAPTER 1 The Radiological Eye

Page 13 For a reproduction of Röntgen's first X-Rays, see C. Singer & E. A. Underwood, *A Short History of Medicine*, 2nd edn, London, Oxford University Press, 1962, pp. 374–76. The first X-Ray for clinical purposes was carried out by Alan Archibald Campbell Swinton in London, in January 1896.
Page 14 See R. & E. Brecher, *The Rays: A History of Radiology in the United States and Canada*, Baltimore, Williams and Wilkins, 1969, for the introduction of radiology into the New World. A month after its introduction, in February 1896, the first side-effects were reported from Nashville, Tennessee, and throughout that year other reports of side-effects began to accumulate.
Page 15 Susan Sontag, *On Photography*, Harmondsworth, Penguin, 1973.
Page 16 Mrs Alec Tweedie, *Mexico as I Saw It*, London, Hurst and Blackett, 1902, pp. 215–16. The festival is still the same today. See *Mexico: The Day of the Dead*, Chloë Sayer (ed.), London, Redstone Press, 1990. Illustrations of *El Dia de los Muertos* feature prominently in the work of the famous Mexican popular artist José Guadalupe Posada, one of the inspirations for the later work of the muralist Diego Rivera.
Page 16 For a textbook of radiology with illustrations of the many forms of X-Ray, see D. Sutton (ed.), *Textbook of Radiology*, 2nd edn, Edinburgh, Churchill Livingstone, 1975.

CHAPTER 2 The Body of Frankenstein's Monster

Page 19 A much shorter version of this paper appeared in 1988 as: Cecil Helman, 'Dr Frankenstein and the Industrial Body', *Anthropology Today*, published by the Royal Anthropological Institute, Vol. 4, No. 3, pp. 14–16.
Page 21 P. M. Jensen, *Boris Karloff and his Films*, New York, A. S. Barnes, 1974.
Page 21 Mary Shelley, *Frankenstein*, New York, Signet Classics, 1965.
Page 21 For the literary and historical background to Mary Shelley's *Frankenstein*, see Radu Florescu, *In Search of Frankenstein*, Boston, New York Graphic Society, 1975. He includes a 'filmography of all Frankenstein films from 1910 till 1976, and also discusses Paracelsus' homunculus, the artificial man of Albertus Magnus, and other early automata.
Page 22 Brian Aldiss, in *The Observer Magazine*, 5 May 1980, p. 71, calls *Frankenstein* 'a diseased creation myth'.
Page 22 In their book *The Wise Wound*, London, Gollancz, 1978, Penelope Shuttle and Peter Redgrove use the term 'Barren' Frankenstein.

Notes

Page 22 The quote is from Drake Douglas, *Horrors*, London, John Baker, 1967.

Page 22 For a discussion of the Golem legends, see Gershom G. Scholem, *On the Kaballah and Its Symbolism*, New York, Schocken Books, 1969, pp. 158–204. He notes (p.166) the limited nature of the Golem, and that in all the legends the artificial man 'is always lacking in some essential function.' The Hebrew word for earth is 'Adamah', thought to be the etymology of the name 'Adam'.

Page 23 Denis Gifford, *Monsters of the Movies*, London, Carousel, 1977. The films mentioned here are: *Dr Jekyll and Mr Hyde* (1931), *The Island of Lost Souls* (1932), *Doctor X* (1932), *The Mad Monster* (1941), *Dr Strangelove, or How I Learnt to Stop Worrying and Love the Bomb* (1963), and the famous German Expressionist film *The Cabinet of Dr Caligari* (1919).

Page 23 Mary Douglas, in *Natural Symbols* (Harmondsworth, Penguin, pp. 93–112, 1970), discusses the use of the body as a 'natural symbol' through which we interpret social life. 'The physical experience of the body, always modified by the social categories through which it is known, sustains a particular view of society. There is a continual exchange of meanings between the two kinds of bodily experience, so that each reinforces the categories of the other.'

Page 23 Western society is a collection of autonomous individuals, notes the anthropologist Deborah Gordon, and thus we see the body as a collection of individual organs. Deborah R. Gordon, *Magico-Religious Dimensions of Bio-medicine: The Case of the Artificial Heart*, unpublished MS, 1987.

Page 24 The quote is from S. I. Schwartz, G. T. Shires, F. C. Spencer & E. H. Stoner, *Principles of Surgery*, 3rd edn, New York, McGraw Hill, 1979. They use the phrase 'organ harvest' to describe the collection of organs for transplantation from cadavers.

Page 25 K. Cowan, *Implant and Transplant Surgery*, London, John Murray, 1971. A summary of advances in 'spare part' surgery, though much has happened in this field since then.

Page 25 Alvin Toffler, *Future Shock*, London, Pan, 1970, p. 193.

Page 27 Robert Malone's *The Robot Book*, New York, Harcourt Brace Jovanovich, 1978, is an illustrated history of robots and automata, and their portrayal in fiction and film, from the earliest times until today.

Page 28 The term 'neomort' appears in K. Stein, 'Redefining Death', *OMNI*, Vol. 9, No. 12, 1987, p. 58.

CHAPTER 3 The Rise of Germism

Page 29 *The Common Cold: Relief But No Cure*, Department of Health and Human Services, Rockville, Maryland, 1983. HHS Publication No. (FDA) 77–3029. Reprinted from *FDA Consumer*, Sept. 1976.

Page 29 *Germs are a Dirty Business*, Health Education Council, London, Pamphlet HY 16, undated.

Page 31 Susan Sontag, *Illness as Metaphor*, Vintage Books, New York, 1979.

Page 31 For a discussion of the history of microbiology, see C. Singer & E. A. Underwood, *A Short History of Medicine*, 2nd edn, Oxford University Press, 1962, pp. 126, 326–41 & 352–62. Louis Pasteur (1822–1895) demonstrated in 1859 that the air contained living organisms and published his *Memoire sur les corpuscles organisés qui existent dans l'atmosphere* ('Memoir on the Organized Bodies which exist in the Air') in 1861. Robert Koch (1843–1910) demonstrated the Tubercle bacillus in 1882, and the Cholera bacillus in 1883. Theodore Klebs (1834–1913) described the Diphtheria Bacillus (corynebacterium diphtheriae) in 1883/84. Joseph Lister (1827–1912), a surgeon, in 1865 realized from the writings of Pasteur that wound infection was not due to 'putrefaction', but to 'a fermentation . . . caused by the products of growth of microscopic organisms borne by the air'. He 'cleaned' the air by Carbolic spray. Later, *a*sepsis superseded *anti*sepsis, based on the work of William Macewen (1848–1924), a surgeon of Glasgow, who began in the 1870s to boil all his instruments and dressings.

Page 32 See my own paper: Cecil G. Helman, '"Feed a Cold, Starve a Fever"': Folk Models of Infection in an English Suburban Community, and their Relation to Medical Treatment', *Culture, Medicine and Psychiatry*, 2, 1978, pp. 107–37.

Page 34 Faye Ainscow, 'Weary search for a suitable psychoanalyst', *The Independent*, London, Tuesday 25 October 1988, p. 15.

Page 35 Paul Ehrlich, Address delivered September 1906, in *The Collected Papers of Paul Ehrlich*, F. Himmelwert (ed.), London, Pergamon, 1960.

Page 36 Mary Douglas, *Purity and Danger*, Harmondsworth, Penguin, 1966, p. 48. Her book deals with cultural notions of pollution, holiness and purity.

Page 38 For a discussion of the *daemones*, see Peter Brown, 'Sorcery, Demons, and the Rise of Christianity', in *Witchcraft Confessions and Accusations*, Mary Douglas (ed.), London, Tavistock, 1970, pp. 17–45. The quote is from E. Dawes & E. & N. H. Baynes, *Three Byzantine Saints*, Oxford, Blackwell, 1948, p. xii. See also *The Oxford Classical Dictionary*, M. Cary *et al.* (eds), London, Oxford University Press, 1966, p. 743, for a discussion of the eleventh-century Greek writer, Michael Psellus of Constantinople (1018–78/9) who wrote *De Operatione Daemonum* (The Operations of Daemones).

Page 40 Marion Starkey, *The Devil in Massachusetts*, London, Trust Books, 1963. For the European witch-hunts see H. R. Trevor-Roper, *The European Witch-Craze of the 16th and 17th Centuries*, Harmondsworth, Penguin, 1969.

Page 40 See Marion Starkey, *op. cit.*

Page 41 I. M. Lewis, *Ecstatic Religion*, Harmondsworth, Penguin, 1971. 'These malign pathogenic spirits are regarded as being extremely captious and capricious . . . They are not concerned with man's behaviour to man . . . they have no interest in defending the moral code of society, and those who succumb to their unwelcome attentions are morally blameless.'

Page 42 See C. Singer & E. A. Underwood, *op. cit.*

Page 43 See *Medical Knowledge: Doubt and Certainty*, Milton Keynes, Open

University Press, 1985, pp. 35–8, for a discussion of the role of epidemics in human history, including the destruction of the Aztec and Incan empires – most dramatic instance of the impact of infectious diseases on human history – and the major epidemics in Europe: the Great Plague of London of 1665–6, the other plagues in the seventeenth and eighteenth centuries, up to the Marseille and Toulon epidemics of 1720–22. The Flagellant movement took place during the Black Death, in 1348–9.

Page 44 The eye-witness account of Guy de Chauliac is reproduced in *The Autobiography of Science*, Forest Jay Moulton and Justus J. Schifferes (eds), New York, Doubleday, Doran and Company, 1945, pp. 38–40.

Page 44 Susan Sontag, *op. cit.* p. 58. The quote from Hitler, in 1919, is on p. 80.

Page 45 The Plague bacillus was discovered in 1894, the role of the flea emerged only in 1898.

Page 46 See Andrew Britton, 'AIDS apocalyptic metaphor', *New Statesman*, 15 March 1985. He notes the 'contagious' image of homosexuality in the media coverage of AIDS.

CHAPTER 4 Half-Green, Half-Black

Page 48 See my own book: *Culture, Health and Illness: An Introduction for Health Professionals*, 2nd edn, Wright/Butterworths, 1990. See Chapter 8, 'Culture and Pharmacology', and Chapter 11, 'Cultural Aspects of Stress', for a discussion of the placebo and nocebo phenomena.

Page 49 For the placebo effect in medicine, see A. K. Shapiro, 'The Placebo Effect in the History of Medical Treatment: Implications for Psychiatry', *American Journal of Psychiatry*, Vol. 116, 1959, pp. 298–304; H. Benson & M. D. Epstein, 'The Placebo Effect: A Neglected Asset in the Care of Patients', *Journal of the American Medical Association*, Vol. 232, 1975, pp. 1225–7; and H. M. Adler & V. O. Hammett, 'The Doctor–Patient Relationship Revisited: An Analysis of the Placebo Effect', *Annals of Internal Medicine*, Vol. 78, 1973, pp. 595–8. In J. D. Levine, N. C. Gordon & H. L. Fields, 'The Mechanism of Placebo Analgesia', *Lancet*, Vol. 2, 1978, pp. 654–7, they suggest that pain-relief from placebos is due to the secretion by the brain of 'endorphins', or other endogenous opiates. For a philosophical perspective on placebos, see Howard Brody, *Placebos and the Philosophy of Medicine: Clinical, Conceptual, and Ethical Issues*, Chicago, University of Chicago Press, 1986.

Page 49 K. Schapira *et al.*, 'Study on the Effects of Tablet Colour in the Treatment of Anxiety States', *British Medical Journal*, 2, 1970, pp. 446–9; A. Branthwaite & P. Cooper, 'Analgesic Effects of Branding in Treatment of Headaches', *British Medical Journal*, 282, 1981, pp. 1576–8; M. Jefferys, J. H. F. Brotherston & A. Cartwright, 'Consumption of Medicines on a Working-class Housing Estate', *British Journal of Preventive and Social Medicine*, 14, 1960, pp. 64–76.

Page 49 New drugs are tested by the so-called 'double-blind trial', whereby one group of subjects are given the drug, while another group with the same medical condition are given a placebo identical in appearance to the drug. To exclude the placebo effect of either the patient's or the researcher's belief in the drug, neither knows – until after the tests have ended – who was given a placebo, and who was given the pharmacologically 'real' drug. In these trials, usually about one-third of the placebo group actually recover from their symptoms or medical condition. See Gordon Claridge, *Drugs and Human Behaviour*, London, Allen Lane, 1970. Chapter 2 includes a summary of research into the placebo effect. For psychological dependency on placebos, see the Editorial in the *Lancet*, 2, 1972, pp. 122–3.

Page 50 For a history of Mesmer, see Louis Rose, *Faith Healing*, Harmondsworth, Penguin, 1974, pp. 52–7. For a description of Phineas Parkhurst Quimby (1802–66), and other famous faith healers, see pp. 61–4. Another famous Quimby statement was: 'Disease is false reasoning. False reasoning is sickness and Death.'

Page 54 For a study of the symbolic aspects of tranquillizers, sleeping tablets and other psychotropic drugs, see C. G. Helman, '"Tonic", "Fuel", and "Food": Social and Symbolic Aspects of the Long-term Use of Psychotrophic Drugs', *Social Science and Medicine*, Vol. 15B, 1981, pp. 521–33.

Page 54 For a discussion of 'voodoo death' or 'hex death', see Barbara W. Lex, 'Voodoo Death: New Thoughts on an Old Explanation', in *Culture, Disease and Healing*, David Landy (ed.), New York, Macmillan, 1977, pp. 327–31; and Claude Lévi-Strauss, *Structural Anthropology*, New York, Anchor Books, 1967, pp. 161–2. The classic physiological explanation for voodoo death was given by W. Cannon in his paper, 'Voodoo Death', *American Anthropologist*, Vol. 44, 1942, pp. 169–81. He argued that it was due to over-activity of the sympathetic nervous system – the 'flight or fight' response – in a situation where the individual is culturally immobilized, and prevented from doing either. This may possibly cause arrhythmias of the heart, or other dangerous physiological changes.

CHAPTER 5 The Premenstrual Werewolf

Page 58 Paul Chandler, 'Harley St alert on PMT women. GPs are warned: Treat "animal" syndrome seriously', *Doctor*, November 19, 1981. In the same article is a report from Norwich Crown Court about a divorcee who killed her lover and was given a 12-month conditional discharge, and set free. She too had been suffering from Premenstrual Tension, and pleaded guilty to manslaughter with 'diminished responsibility'. The term 'Premenstrual Tension' was coined by an American gynaecologist in 1931: i.e. Robert Frank, 'The Hormonal Causes of Premenstrual Tension', *Archives of Neurology and Psychiatry*, 1931, 26, p. 1053. According to Dr Katharina Dalton in *The Premenstrual Syndrome*, London, Heinemann, 1964, it is 'the commonest endocrine disorder', and is associated with increased marital disharmony, increased sexual activity, accidents, crimes of violence, shoplifting and suicide attempts. For a history of the imagery of menstruation see J. Delaney, M. J. Lupton &

Notes

E. Toth, *The Curse: A Cultural History of Menstruation*, New York, Dutton, 1976.

Page 60 See *Encyclopaedia Britannica, Micropaedia*, Vol. X, 15th edn, 1974, p. 617, for definition of a Werewolf as 'a man who turns into a wolf at night and devours animals, people, or corpses, but returns to human form by day. Some werewolves change shape involuntarily, under the influence of a full moon. If wounded in wolf form, the wound will show in his human form and may lead to his detection.'

Page 60 For a description of the *fylgja*, and the roots of werewolf myths in Teutonic mythology, as well as the story of Sigmund and Sinfjöth, see the *New Larousse Encyclopaedia of Mythology*, London, Hamlyn, 1977, pp. 277–8.

Page 61 Most 'Werewolf' and 'Cat' films are listed in Les Daniels, *Fear: A History of Horror in the Mass Media*, London, Paladin, 1977; and in David Pirie, *A Heritage of Horror: The English Gothic Cinema 1946–1972*, New York, Avon Books, 1973; and in other books. Such films include: *The Wolf Man* (1941), *The Werewolf of London* (1935), *The Cat and the Canary* (1939), *The Mad Monster* (1941), *The Undying Monster* (1942), *The Cat People* (1942), *Frankenstein meets the Wolfman* (1943), *Curse of the Cat People* (1944), *Jungle Captive* (1944), *Cry of the Werewolf* (1944), *Catman of Paris* (1946), *The Werewolf* (1956), *Cat Girl* (1957), *I was a Teenage Werewolf* (1957), *Island of Lost Souls* (1932), *Curse of the Werewolf* (1961), *Werewolf in a Girls' Dormitory* (1961), *Beauty and the Beast* (1963), *Werewolves on Wheels* (1971), *Werewolf of Washington* (1973), *Legend of the Werewolf* (1975), *An American Werewolf in London* (1981).

Page 62 Many of the cinematic man-animals and the magical transformations from man to hybrid animal-man or animal-woman are described in Denis Gifford, *Monsters of the Movies*, London, Carousel, 1977.

Page 63 See the *New Larousse Encyclopaedia of Mythology*, London, Hamlyn, 1977, for descriptions of many of these mythological creatures from ancient Greece, Egypt, Assyria, Babylonia and India, as well as the Teutonic werewolf.

Page 64 See Malcolm Ruel, 'Were-animals and the Introverted Witch', in *Witchcraft Confessions and Accusations*, Mary Douglas (ed.), London, Tavistock, 1970, pp. 33–5, for a description of Banyang beliefs about were-animals.

Page 65 The quotations are from a 1566 witchcraft trial. See Alan Macfarlane, 'Witchcraft in Tudor and Stuart Essex', in *Witchcraft Confessions and Accusations*, Mary Douglas (ed.), London, Tavistock, 1970.

Page 66 *The Epic of Gilgamesh*, translated by N. K. Sandars, Harmondsworth, Penguin Books, 1960; and also the *New Larousse Encyclopaedia of Mythology*.

Page 66 Descriptions of the *utokoloshe* and the *uthikoloshe* are in J. A. Brandford, *Dictionary of South African English*, Oxford University Press, 1978.

Page 67 The two classic papers on the anthropology of hair are C. R. Hallpike's 'Social Hair', in *MAN*, 4 (n.s.), 1969, pp. 256–64, and Edmund Leach's 'Magical Hair' in the *Journal of the Royal Anthropological Institute*, 88, part 2, July–Dec 1958, pp. 147–64.

Page 68 Jeremiah, Chapter 7, Verse 29.

Page 68 These colloquial uses of 'hair' appear in the *Penguin Dictionary of Historical Slang*, Eric Partridge (ed.), Harmondsworth, Penguin, 1972, pp. 416–17.

Page 69 Genesis, Chapter 25, Verse 27, and Chapter 27, Verse 11.

Page 69 George Fox's experience is related in *The Weaker Vessel* by Antonia Fraser, Mandarin Publishers, 1989, pp. 3, 526.

Page 70 The quote from Charles Darwin is reproduced in *The Woman's History of the World* by Rosalind Miles, Paladin Books, 1989, p. 227.

Page 72 Bruno Bettelheim, *The Uses of Enchantment*, New York, Vintage, 1977, pp. 166–83.

Page 73 *The Company of Wolves*, 1985. Directed by Neil Jordan, and based on a story by Angela Carter.

Page 73 Robert Eisler, *Man into Wolf: An Anthropological Interpretation of Sadism, Masochism, and Lycanthropy*, London, Routledge and Kegan Paul, 1951. He uses the phrase 'a big dame hunter' on page 227. After WW1 and WW2, para-military groups in Germany were formed called 'Werewolfs' to oppose the Allied occupation forces (page 33).

Page 75 The story of Peter Stubb, and other sixteenth- and seventeenth-century werewolves, is told by Brian Ward in 'Werewolves: a culture-bound psychosis', *World Medicine*, 30 May 1973, pp. 43–55.

Page 75 P. E. Keck, H. G. Pope, J. I. Hudson, S. L. McElroy & A. R. Kulick, 'Lycanthropy: alive and Well in the Twentieth Century', *Psychological Medicine*, 18, 1988, pp. 113–20. Diagnosis of lycanthropy should include at least one of the following criteria: '(1) The individual reported verbally, during intervals of lucidity or retrospectively, that he or she was a particular animal. (2) The individual behaved in a manner reminiscent of a particular animal, i.e. howling, growling, crawling on all fours.' In the *Encyclopaedia Britannica, Micropaedia*, Vol. VI, 1974, p. 409, 'Lycanthropy' is defined as 'a psychotic state in which the patient believes he is a wolf or some other non-human animal'. It is supposed to be more common among peoples who believe in reincarnation.

Page 77 Mary Douglas, *Natural Symbols*, Harmondsworth, Penguin, 1973, p. 93.

Page 77 In *The Wise Wound: Menstruation and Everywoman*, London, Gollancz, 1978, Penelope Shuttle and Peter Redgrove suggest that men's emotional reaction to menstruation is part terror, part desire, of becoming a woman. Furthermore, 'men have always feared and been fascinated by female mysteries, and have attempted to annex them, and to minimize the contribution of women.' They point out how in some tribes, male rites of puberty circumcision mimic the onset of menstruation, with blood spilt by a knife, and not by nature.

Page 78 The statements by Father Jerome and Bishop Isidore of Seville, and other early theological views of women, are quoted in *A History of their Own:*

Women in Europe from Prehistory to the Present, by Bonnie S. Anderson and Judith P. Zinsser, Penguin Books, 1988, pp. 77–90.

Page 78 See Mary Chamberlain, *Old Wives' Tales*, London, Virago, 1981, for traditional English beliefs about the polluting power of menstruation, especially in the preparation of food.

Page 79 Stanislas Klossowski de Rola, *Alchemy: The Secret Art*, London, Thames and Hudson, 1973.

CHAPTER 6 The Medusa Machine

Page 83 Illustrations of some of these eigthteenth-century automata appear in Robert Malone's *The Robot Book*, New York, Harcourt Brace Jovanovich, 1978.

Page 83 The most famous automaton-makers were the Frenchman Jacques de Vaucanson (1709–1782), and the Swiss Pierre Jacquet-Droz (1721–90) and his son Henri-Louis (1753–1791). Vaucanson's automata were shown in England in 1742, and elsewhere in Europe. In 1782, King George III ordered Jacquet-Droz to make a copy of the 'Writing Boy', as a gift to the Emperor of China.

Page 84 Radu Florescu, *In Search of Frankenstein*, Boston, New York Graphic Society, 1975. He describes Mary Shelley's travels through Europe, including her visit to Neuchâtel.

Page 84 Several automata of Pierre and Henri-Louis Jacquet-Droz are preserved in the Musée d'Art et d'Histoire, Neuchâtel, Switzerland.

Page 85 See Marshal McLuhan's, *Understanding Media: The Extensions of Man*, London, Sphere Books, 1967, for a discussion of the effect of the new communications media on contemporary culture.

Page 86 *The New Larousse Encyclopaedia of Mythology*, London, Hamlyn, 1977, p. 183. The three Gorgon sisters were Stheno, Euryale and Medusa. Instead of teeth they had the tusks of wild boars, hands of bronze, golden wings on their shoulders, with locks of writhing serpents; 'whoever dared to look them in the face was instantly turned to stone.' Of the three, only Medusa was mortal, and she was killed and then decapitated by the hero Perseus, after which he fled on Pegasus' back, carrying her head, and pursued by the other two Gorgons.

Page 87 Cecil Helman, *Culture, Health and Illness: an Introduction for Health Professionals*, 2nd edn, John Wright, 1990. See Chapter 2, pp. 11–22, 'Cultural Conceptions of Anatomy and Physiology'. For an illustration of the 'plumbing model' of anatomy, see A. Kleinman, L. Eisenberg & B. Good, 'Clinical Lessons from Anthropologic and Cross-cultural Research', *Annals of Internal Medicine*, Vol. 88, 1978, pp. 251–8.

Page 88 Sherry Turkle, *The Second Self: Computers and the Human Spirit*, London, Granada, 1984.

Page 88 Frank George, *Man the Machine*, London, Granada, 1979, a study of the new generation of advanced computers, and their implications for future society.

Page 91 In *Zen and the Art of Motorcycle Maintenance*, Ealing, Corgi, 1974, Robert M. Pirsig notes how *all* machines tell us something about the minds of their creators, especially the system of thought and organization that they are employing. Even 'the motorcycle is primarily a mental phenomenon'.

CHAPTER 7 A Bridge of Organs

Page 94 With some fictionalization, this story is based on a real clinical case that I encountered some years ago.

Page 96 The Munchausen Syndrome was first described by R. Asher: 'Munchausen Syndrome', *Lancet*, i, 1951, pp. 339–41. Its three classical criteria were: exaggerated symptoms, 'factitious' physical signs, and the tendency to wander between hospitals.

Page 100 Roland Barthes described the mythological significance of Einstein's brain in his essay 'The Brain of Einstein' in *Mythologies*, London, Granada, 1981, pp. 68–70.

Page 100 For a description of the cult of devotion to the Sacred Heart, see N. Boyadjian, *The Heart: its History, its Symbolism, its Iconography and its Diseases*, Antwerp, Esco Books, 1980, pp. 28–31. Christ appeared in human form to St Lutgarde d'Aywiers: 'What asketh thou of me?' he said to her. 'I wish for your heart,' she replied. 'And I desire thy heart even more.'

Page 101 *King Lear*, Act 5, Scene 3.

Page 102 'The Tell-Tale Heart' in *Edgar Allan Poe: Selected Writings*, Paul Galloway (ed.), Harmondsworth, Penguin English Library, 1967.

Page 102 For a cautiously critical review of the claims of Phrenology, and the early ideas of Neurology, see the article 'Phrenology' in *The Encyclopaedia Britannica*, 1910–1911 edn, Vol. XXI, pp. 534–41.

Page 104 See the Open University course book, *Medical Knowledge: Doubt and Certainty*, Open University Press, 1985, pp. 59–92, for a discussion of the reasons for the 'epidemic of hysterectomies'. They suggest it may be linked to traditional notions of hysteria as unique to women and originating in the womb – thus the name *furor uterinus* traditionally given to the condition. They also suggest hysterical behaviour may be a reaction to women's lack of power. Some studies have shown that hysterical female patients still have an excessive rate of hysterectomies; see M. E. Cohen, E. Robins, J. J. Purtell, M. W. Altmann & D. E. Reid, 'Excessive Surgery in Hysteria', *Journal of the American Medical Association*, Vol. 151, 1953, pp. 977–986. The concept of the 'wandering womb' and the quote from Jean Libault are on page 90 of *Medical Knowledge*.

Page 104 For a discussion of the British and their bowels, see Lynn Payer, *Medicine and Culture*, London, Victor Gollancz, 1989, pp. 116–18. The French obsession with their livers, apparently originating in the Middle Ages, is described on pages 56–61.

Page 105 Eric J. Cassell, 'Disease as an "It": Concepts of Disease Revealed by Patients' Presentation of Symptoms', *Social Science and Medicine*, Vol. 10, 1976, pp. 143–6.

Notes

Page 106 These quotations and those on page 107 are from my own research, carried out at Harvard Medical School in Boston in 1983/84, and published as: Cecil Helman, 'Psyche, Soma and Society: The Social Construction of Psychosomatic Disorders', in *Culture, Medicine and Psychiatry*, Vol. 9, 1985, pp. 1–26.

Page 109 Herbert Weiner, *9 Mystics: The Kabbala Today*, New York, Collier, 1969.

Page 109 See Nancy Scheper-Hughes & Margaret M. Lock, 'The Mindful Body: A Prolegomenon to Future Work in Medical Anthropology', *Medical Anthropology Quarterly* (New Series), Vol. 1, No. 1, 1987, pp. 6–41. 'In ancient Chinese cosmology,' they write, 'the emphasis is on balance and resonance; in Western cosmology, on tension and contradiction.' They also discuss in more detail the soul-beliefs of Zinancantan and the Cuna Indians of Panama. Also see Evon Vogt, *Zinancantan: A Mayan Community in the Highlands of Chiapas*, Cambridge, Massachusetts, Belknap Press of Harvard University Press, 1969.

Page 109 See Charles Singer & E. Ashworth Underwood, *A Short History of Medicine*, 2nd edn, London, Oxford University Press, 1962, for an outline of Hippocratic and Galenic theories of physiology. Galen lived from c.129–c.200 AD.

Page 110 Ayurvedic Medicine is described by Ganath Obeyesekere, 'The Theory and Practice of Ayurvedic Medicine', *Culture, Medicine and Psychiatry*, 1, 1977, pp. 155–81.

Page 110 See Alexander Macdonald, *Acupuncture*, London, Unwin, 1984, for a brief introduction to the Yellow Emperor's *Classic of Internal Medicine*.

CHAPTER 8 The Dissecting Room

Page 115 *Ellis's Anatomy*, J. A. Keen (ed.) 2nd edn, Pietermaritzburg, University of Natal Press, 1957.

Page 118 See J. L. Thornton & C. Reeves, *Medical Book Illustration: A Short History*, Cambridge, Oleander Press, 1983, for an illustrated outline of dissection art, including Vesalius, Leonardo, Dürer and others.

Page 118 Elmer Belt, *Leonardo the Anatomist*, Lawrence, Kansas, University of Kansas Press, 1955.

Page 118 The illustrations of Vesalius, including the famous *de humani corporis fabrica*, are well reproduced in J. B. & C. D. O'Malley, *The Anatomical Drawings of Andreas Vesalius*, New York, Bonanza Books, 1982.

Page 119 The first coloured anatomical illustrations in Europe appear in the book *Mythologie complete en couleur et grandeur naturelle*, Jacques Fabian Gautier-d'Agoty, published in Paris in 1746.

Page 119 Robert Knox, *Great Artists and Great Anatomists: A Biographical and Philosophical Study*, London, John Van Voorst, 1852.

Page 119 *Gray's Anatomy*. First Edition by Henry Gray in 1857/8.

CHAPTER 9 A Time of the Heart

Page 124 Some of the ideas in this chapter are from my own paper: 'Heart Disease and the Cultural Construction of Time: The Type A Behaviour Pattern as a Western Culture-Bound Syndrome', *Social Science and Medicine*, Vol. 25, No. 9, 1987, pp. 969–79.

Page 126 In their 1959 paper, Friedman and Rosenman describe the six core features of the Type A Behaviour Pattern as: (1) an intense, sustained drive to achieve self-selected but usually poorly defined goals, (2) a profound eagerness to compete, (3) a persistent desire for recognition and advancement, (4) a continuous involvement in 'multiple and diverse functions' constantly subject to deadlines, (5) a tendency to accelerate the rate of many physical and mental functions, and (6) an extraordinary mental and physical alertness.

Page 127 Some of the classic papers on the Type A Behaviour Pattern (TABP) are: M. Friedman and R. H. Rosenman, 'Association of Specific Behaviour Pattern with Blood and Cardiovascular Findings', *Journal of the American Medical Association,* Vol. 169, 1959, pp. 1286–96; R. H. Rosenman, R. H. Friedman, R. Straus, M. Wurm, R. Kositchek, W. Hahn & N. T. Wethessen, 'A Predictive Study of Coronary Heart Disease: The Western Collaborative Group Study', *Journal of the American Medical Association*, 189, 1964, pp. 15–22; *Coronary-Prone Behavior*, T. H. Dembrowski *et al.* (eds), New York, Springer, 1978, pp. 199–205; R. Gibbs, *Lifestyle and Coronary Heart Disease*, London, Macmillan, 1979; V. A. Price, *Type A Behavior Pattern: A Model for Research and Practice*, New York, Academic Press, 1983.

Page 129 Edward T. Hall, *The Dance of Life: The Other Dimension of Time*, New York, Anchor Press, 1984.

Page 130 See Joseph Needham, 'Time and Knowledge in China and the West', in *The Voices of Time*, J. T. Fraser (ed.), London, Allen Lane, 1966, pp. 92–135.

Page 130 E. Jacques, in *The Form of Time*, London, Heinemann, 1982, noted that our civilization is characterized by an unconscious 'sense of temporal directionality', reinforced through our conceptualization of time by the use of spatial metaphors.

Page 131 See Marie-Louise Von Franz, *Time, Rhythm and Repose*, Thames and Hudson, London, 1978, for a description of Western and non-Western forms of time.

Page 131 See Christopher Rawlence (ed.), *About Time*, London, Jonathan Cape, 1985, for an excellent book on the nature of time, including the history of British time and its relationship to industry and work.

Page 132 See R. H. Knapp & J. T. Garbutt, 'Time Imagery and the Achievement Motive', *J. Person.*, Vol. 26, 1982, pp. 32–6. As they put it: 'it was in just those North European cultures which fostered entrepreneurship, the emphasis on achievement motivation, and the rise of capitalism, that time pieces first helped establish the rise of a time-monitored industrialism.'

Page 134 J. T. Fraser, 'Comments on Time, Process, and Achievement', and also 'The Study of Time', in *The Voices of Time*, J. T. Fraser (ed.), London, Allen Lane, 1966.

Page 134 Max Weber, *The Protestant Ethic and the Spirit of Capitalism*, London, Allen and Unwin, 1948. This was a reprint of the original essay that appeared in German in 1904/5 as *Die protestantische Ethik und der Geist des Kapitalismus.*

Page 135 The essay is reprinted in *Works of the late Doctor Benjamin Franklin*, London, Robinson, 1794, pp. 60–5.

Page 135 See M. Friedman & R. H. Rosenman, 'Association of Specific Behavior Pattern with Blood and Cardiovascular Findings', *Journal of the American Medical Association*, Vol. 169, 1959, pp. 1286–96; and R. H. Rosenman, 'Role of Type A Behavior Pattern in the Pathogenesis of Ischaemic Heart Disease, and Modification for Prevention,' *Advances in Cardiology*, Vol. 25, 1978, pp. 35–46.

Page 136 Sir William Osler, *Lectures on Angina Pectoris and Allied States*, New York, Appleton, 1897.

Page 136 Dr Eric J. Cassell, *The Healer's Art*, Philadelphia, Lippincott, 1976, pp. 41–2.

Page 136 Some of the medical arguments against the claims of the Type A Behaviour model are summarized in M. G. Marmot, 'Stress, Social and Cultural Variations in Heart Disease', *Journal of Psychosomatic Research*, 27, 1983, pp. 377–84. He points out that Type A Behaviour does not follow the distribution of CHD in the population: e.g. in the Whitehall study, lower income men had a greater risk of CHD, but a lower prevalence of Type A Behaviour, while in the Framingham study working women had less heart disease than men, but an equal prevalence of the TABP. The exact mechanism whereby TABP causes CHD is still not known (see R. H. Rosenman, 'Role of Type A Behavior Pattern in the Pathogenesis of Ischaemic Heart Disease, and Modification for Prevention', *Advances in Cardiology*, 25, 1978, pp. 35–46). Also, most studies have been carried out on 'white, middle-class, middle-aged males in the United States': J. B. Cohen, K. A. Matthews & I. Waldron, 'Coronary-prone Behavior: Development and Cultural Considerations', in *Coronary-Prone Behavior*, T. H. Dembrowski *et al.* (eds), New York, Springer, 1978, pp. 184–90.

Page 138 In the study by B. Cowie, 'The Cardiac Patient's Perception of his Heart Attack', *Social Science and Medicine*, Vol. 10, 1976, pp. 87–96, he found that patients recovering from a heart attack (myocardial infarction) in a coronary care unit, engaged in 'retrospective reconstruction' of their own biographies – in such a way that their heart attack was perceived as the obvious outcome of their previous life-style.